CW01217492

Advance praise for *Yoga Saved My Life*

'*Yoga Saved My Life* shows us gently and persuasively that healing the mind is as important as healing the body, and yoga is a great way of doing this.'
Vex King, author of *Good Vibes, Good Life* and *Healing is the New High*

'During this very ugly moment in global history, we all need as much support as possible. Thankfully, Sasha Bates has gifted us with a magnificent jewel, exploring the physical and psychological benefits of yoga and so much more besides. This extremely readable and engaging book offers essential life-saving wisdom and calm.'
Professor Brett Kahr, Senior Fellow, Tavistock Institute of Medical Psychology, London, and Visiting Professor of Psychoanalysis and Mental Health, Regent's University London.

'Such a wonderfully enjoyable – and practical – book. A lovely guided voice making sense in a crowded space.'
Liz Earle, MBE

'Sasha takes everyday issues of modern life – stress, anxiety, depression, insecurity, overwhelm – and clearly unpacks them psychotherapeutically while revealing how the practice of yoga can help us grow in tolerance, agency, purpose, and compassion.'
Sandra Gillespie, Somatic Therapist, London, UK

'Sasha demystifies yoga and gives a refreshing antidote to the off-putting public face that yoga sometimes presents.'
Karen Russell, senior hatha yoga teacher, and adaptive and sports yoga teacher.

Also by Sasha Bates

Languages of Loss
A Grief Companion

For my mother, Ellie Bates

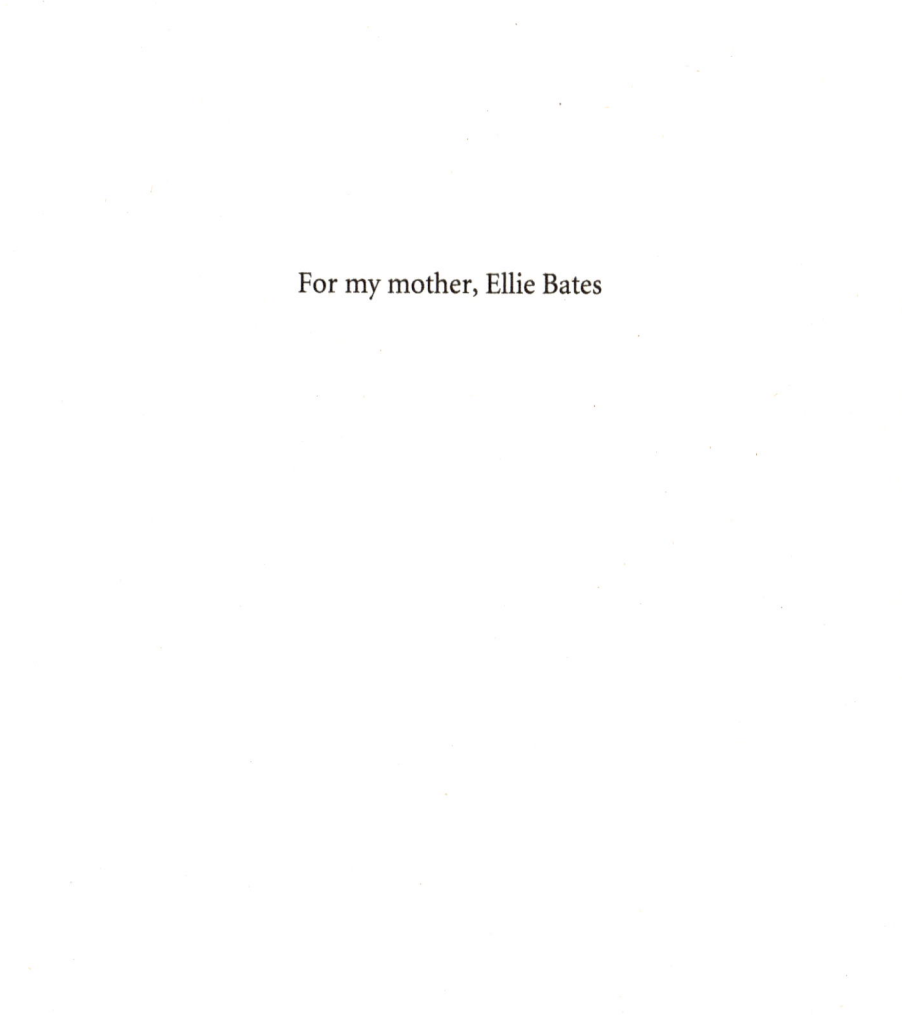

Yoga Saved My Life

SASHA BATES

foreword by **LEE WATSON** of **FIERCE CALM**

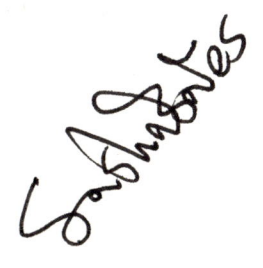

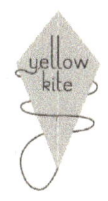

yellow kite

The information in this book is not intended to constitute medical advice, nor is it intended to replace the advice given to you by your doctor or other health professional. If you are not sure whether the yoga practices are suitable for you, or if you have any medical condition, you are advised to consult with your doctor, yoga teacher or other health and fitness professional before starting. The author and publisher disclaim any liability directly or indirectly from the use of the material in this book by any person.

First published in Great Britain in 2022 by Yellow Kite
An Imprint of Hodder & Stoughton
An Hachette UK company

1

Copyright © Sasha Bates 2022
Foreword copyright © Lee Watson 2022

The right of Sasha Bates to be identified as the Author of the Work has been asserted by her in accordance with the Copyright, Designs and Patents Act 1988.

Stories and contributions have been added with permission. Some names have been changed to protect the identity of contributors.

Illustrations by Isobel Tokatly © Hodder & Stoughton

All rights reserved. No part of this publication may be reproduced, stored in a retrieval system, or transmitted, in any form or by any means without the prior written permission of the publisher, nor be otherwise circulated in any form of binding or cover other than that in which it is published and without a similar condition being imposed on the subsequent purchaser.

A CIP catalogue record for this title is available from the British Library

Hardback ISBN 978 1 529 35687 8
eBook ISBN 978 1 529 35688 5
Audiobook 978 1 529 35689 2

Typeset in Minion by Manipal Technologies Limited

Printed and bound in Great Britain by Clays Ltd, Elcograf S.p.A.

Hodder & Stoughton policy is to use papers that are natural, renewable and recyclable products and made from wood grown in sustainable forests. The logging and manufacturing processes are expected to conform to the environmental regulations of the country of origin.

Yellow Kite
Hodder & Stoughton Ltd
Carmelite House
50 Victoria Embankment
London EC4Y 0DZ

www.yellowkitebooks.co.uk

Contents

Foreword by Lee Watson	ix
Introduction	1
Chapter 1: Stressed Out	13
Chapter 2: Anxiety Rules	25
Chapter 3: When Depression Strikes	34
Chapter 4: Find Some Compassion	45
Chapter 5: You Can't Pour From an Empty Cup	59
Chapter 6: Finding Strength	73
Chapter 7: I'm Stuck	82
Chapter 8: Going Into Battle	95
Chapter 9: I Feel Vulnerable	105
Chapter 10: The Swing of the Pendulum	116
Chapter 11: Spinning Out of Control	126
Chapter 12: The Only Way Out Is Through	136
Chapter 13: Take a Leap of Faith	148
Chapter 14: I'm Angry	155
Chapter 15: I Don't Like Conflict	164
Chapter 16: Old Habits Die Hard	176
Chapter 17: The Trauma Response	187
Chapter 18: Is There Anybody Out There?	200
Chapter 19: Shall We Dance?	210
Chapter 20: Dive In	216
Bibliography	220
Notes	230
Acknowledgements	238
About the Author	240

Foreword
by Lee Watson, Fierce Calm

There was a time when, as far as I was concerned, yoga was something that other people did. And when I eventually gave it a go and half-heartedly joined in at the gym, I'll be honest, I thought it was just a 'bit of a stretch'.

I could not have been more wrong.

This book includes numerous personal testimonies from individuals sharing their stories of how their lives have been transformed by yoga, how it helped them heal or learn to live with the various challenges life throws at us. My own yoga story is nowhere near as dramatic as many of theirs but, like many of them, I found out that the more time I spent on a yoga mat, the more it made sense; and the more sense life made off the mat. And that the feeling of calm that crept in at the end of a yoga class was something that became available to me throughout the day. That low-level constant chatter in my head was quieter; I was less anxious, less stressed, more positive and sleeping better.

I wanted everyone to be able to feel that way. I was also aware that not everyone had access to it in the way that I did. I wanted to leverage my privileged position in life to help make yoga available to the people who need it the most.

The more time I spent among the yoga community, the more aware I became of the incredible stories of transformation and recovery supported by this ancient practice. I kept seeing the hashtag #yogasavedmylife. And so Fierce Calm was born, initially as a social media platform featuring the personal stories of those who wanted to share how yoga had helped them.

The stories within these pages are just a snapshot of the thousands shared online, yet, sitting alongside Sasha's unique perspective on how yoga heals, they provide a treasure trove of humanity, of authentic lived experiences that speak of our capacity for resilience, potential to support ourselves and ability to support others. You will see yourself reflected in some of these stories. Each one is a unique opportunity to identify with a life different to our own, yet each also allows us to see our shared humanity in each other.

As we all benefit from hearing each other's stories, as we identify with and endlessly learn from the diverse realities, experiences and resilience of others, our capacity for empathy and compassion grows. And as the thousands of individuals sharing their stories from the heart connected with the hearts of others, they began to come together in the magic of letting others know they are not alone. Friendships and alliances formed. Individuals facing similar issues provided tangible and emotional support for one another. A space that began as individual stories blossomed into a global collective committed to making a difference. The word yoga means *union*, and we have united to be of service to others. A year after our first Instagram post, Fierce Calm organised a global charity fundraiser that saw yoga teachers host classes simultaneously in over 500 locations around the world (from a barn in Hertfordshire to a Scottish mountaintop, a French chateau, a Brazilian beach, studios in Seoul and a lawn in front of the Statue of Liberty).

As a registered non-profit, Fierce Calm now represents a global movement of yoga practitioners from all backgrounds and abilities who want to make the healing potential of yoga accessible to all, while supporting the most vulnerable in society. We provide free yoga classes in shelters and community spaces, for marginalised and vulnerable groups such as refugees, survivors of violence and people facing systemic bias.

Social justice is at the heart of our yoga and we strive to remove all barriers to access and disrupt inequity and the lack of diversity in the wellness space. We offer yoga teacher training scholarships for marginalised or minoritised-ethnicity students, delivered by teachers reflecting these identities. During the pandemic we provided financial support to yoga teachers around the world who found themselves facing hardship. We are conscious that here in the West we've cherry-picked parts of another culture, profiting and benefiting from a profound cultural extraction rooted in colonialism, and we therefore owe a debt of gratitude to the sources of this ancient tradition and strive to honour its roots. In the spirit of taking steps towards reparation, we have fundraised in aid of the fight against Covid in India and supported shelters there, while also providing yoga to South Asian community support groups in the UK.

We were also part of the organising team behind a symposium featuring experts from across the disciplinary spectrum – including medicine, public health and therapeutic yoga – exploring how yoga could enhance resilience and bolster healthcare systems burdened by the Covid-19 crisis. We do not claim that yoga will protect you from a virus, but it is an accessible practice that provides practitioners with ways to manage stress, build resilience and promote healing. As an adjunct therapy to conventional Western medicine, yoga supports the restoration of health and well-being for individuals and healthcare systems suffering the impact of long Covid, contributes to easing the mental health crisis and negative effects of social isolation and assists healthcare workers facing burnout.

This book focuses on individual stories, but when we learn how to take care of ourselves, we are better able to take care of others, our community, of this planet we call home – and when we explore beyond our individual practice and healing journey we all have the power to make the world a better place. Yoga is for everybody. You don't need to be flexible or look like the influencers on social media. The world doesn't need more people who can put their leg behind their head or rock the most expensive leggings; it needs greater kindness, compassion, generosity and empathy. And a practice that encompasses all aspects of yoga beyond the merely physical offers us all of that.

Yoga promotes our capacity to tolerate the challenges of being a human being. It is not a way to bypass life's difficulties, but it does offer us tools to meet them head on, with a fierce dignity and calm. This book shows you how.

Lee Watson,
October 2021

@fierce_calm
www.fierce-calm.com
#yogasavedmylife

Introduction

Yoga saved my life. That's such a bold claim. Yet every day stories pour into the Fierce Calm inbox saying just that: Yoga. Saved. My. Life.

Many of the men and women sharing these stories have been living their lives feeling a little – or a lot – depressed, anxious, angry or chaotic; overtired, overstretched and overwhelmed by their own emotions and the stress of modern life. Some of them talk of feeling out of control, to the point of being in thrall to addictions or post-traumatic stress. Suicidal even. And, they say, yoga may have saved them from all that, transforming their lives in the process.

These claims may seem extraordinary, unbelievable almost, if you think of yoga (as many in the West do tend to) as merely a sequence of exercises to stretch and strengthen your body. It is that, of course, but that is only the tip of a very big iceberg – there is so much more to yoga.

In this book I will use my experience as both psychotherapist and yoga teacher to explore how and why yoga can be so transformative. Because of my long experience with yoga, I don't find it either extraordinary or unbelievable that so many people are making these powerful claims. Because I could say the same of myself. Yoga has saved *my* life, too, on a number of occasions. It has saved me from a life I might have led, a life of stress and overwork, ill health and low mood. I'm not saying I don't sometimes still struggle with those things in my current life – of course I do – but the intensity and frequency are of a completely different flavour from what they would be if I hadn't been doing yoga for thirty years. My world view is different, my relationship with my body is different, the amount of compassion I have – for myself and for others – is different. And all because of my ongoing relationship with yoga.

If I look at this wearing my psychotherapist's hat, I see many parallels. The concerns that bring my clients into therapy are often the same as those that lead people to yoga. And the way in which I work with them as a therapist, helping them to explore, understand and hopefully alleviate these concerns, mirrors the effects that yoga has on me and my students, and that are discussed by the members of Fierce Calm in their stories here.

Some of you reading this book will similarly have your own rich relationship with yoga; for you, I hope I can help you to gain a deeper understanding of why it contributes so much to your life. Others among you may have no experience of yoga but are curious as to why so many of us extol its virtues so loudly, wondering if perhaps it might be something you could try out. My hope is that seasoned yogis and interested onlookers alike will find illumination here, and so feel inspired to deepen their existing knowledge, or be propelled into finding a teacher and embarking on a practice.

Why Do Yoga?

I often hear people say they could never go to a yoga class because they are not flexible enough. That's a bit like saying you couldn't go to a French class because you don't speak French. I can see where this aversion might come from, though – the most visible face of yoga is the one that bombards us with images of lithe, immaculate, athletic gods and goddesses putting their well-toned bodies into mind-boggling poses while sipping kale juice and

Introduction

spouting platitudes in a quasi-spiritual tone. And that can be a very off-putting world to imagine entering.

But those images reflect only one very small facet of yoga – and a very modern and a very Western one at that. In fact, yoga's history stretches back to the India of about five millennia ago when movement was barely mentioned. The practice has evolved and adapted over time. The active, postural aspect came on the scene only relatively recently and is but one element of a far broader holistic practice – a practice that is deeply steeped in a philosophy espousing a way of living more harmoniously.

Harmoniously with what, though? Well, yoga actually means *union* and that can refer to the harmonious union between many elements – mind and body, internal and external, ground and sky, masculine and feminine, matter and anti-matter. Union within our own selves and union with other selves.

In case this is already all starting to sound a bit too other-worldly, let's bring it back to Earth and look at the kind of things that people from the Fierce Calm community say they get from yoga. What habits, behaviours and issues has yoga helped them to grapple with – to the point of leading them to that huge claim: 'yoga saved my life'? What can hearing their experiences offer you, whether you are contemplating coming to yoga for the first time, or whether you already have a long-standing practice?

The stories we are going to hear are heartbreaking yet hopeful and offer a glimpse into how we in the West seek our own ways of living harmoniously. Stories told by people like Terri-Ann, who found that yoga gave her the skills to manage overwhelming emotions without having to turn to alcohol; Charlie, whose discovery of yoga got him away from the tough-guy image his childhood had made him think was his destiny; and Brienna, who found comfort and support within the yoga community, and on her yoga mat, after the death of her brother.

We will hear about the people who, through doing yoga, feel stronger and more resilient when they had been feeling weak and vulnerable; how those who had felt trapped by their own rigidity became more flexible – literally, emotionally and metaphorically. We'll hear from people who went from being constantly exhausted and aching to finding energy and enthusiasm and rediscovering the enjoyment of movement, realising their bodies could be a source of joy instead of disgust and pain; people who came to trust in themselves better as their self-awareness and self-knowledge deepened, people who have become less reactive in arguments, flying off the handle less often, bursting into tears less often, becoming more able to see things from multiple viewpoints. We will hear how relationships have improved, connections deepened, how observational skills have sharpened, scattered minds have become more focused, people have been able to get things done more quickly and efficiently. The list goes on.

Other stories tell how yoga has helped people cope with serious alcoholism and other addictions, as well as with eating disorders, depression, anxiety, grief, post-traumatic stress and more.

For me, when a combination of a stressful job and painful relationship break-up in my early twenties led to months of insomnia and depression, discovering yoga enabled me to regain the ability to sleep, helped me balance out a severely dysregulated nervous system, and led me to rediscover parts of myself that had got lost along the way. My relationship with yoga adapted over the next thirty years, coming to my aid in all sorts of situations, and deepening my self-knowledge in many different ways. But when my husband died unexpectedly three years ago it truly did feel like yoga saved me. This was twofold; first, with the help of yoga friends and teachers I was able to learn to

Introduction

stand on my own two feet and find myself on solid ground again. And second, after thirty years of practice, the lessons of yoga had been absorbed into my very being so fully that I was able to draw on them, fall back on them, even in my darkest hour. From the depths of my grief, I was able to make use of the habits and knowledge and self-regulating mechanisms that had become so embedded.

How to Use This Book

This book is going to explore some of these powerful outcomes of yoga. But it's important for you to know that this is less a 'how-to-do-it' and more of a 'why-would-I-want-to-and-how-does-it-work?' book. The practicalities of getting yourself into physical postures are really just a route to accessing a different way of experiencing yourself. They are the tip of an iceberg, a conduit into self-exploration, offering different ways of feeling, tolerating and understanding yourself. So, I will refer to postures and their benefits, but what I'm <u>not</u> going to do is tell you how to do them. You will need to find a good teacher to show you the postures, to explain safe alignment and sequencing of those postures and work with you to make sure you are not hurting yourself.

What I <u>am</u> going to do is show you how yoga can be transformational, reveal how closely aligned it is to what we do in psychotherapy and illuminate why its benefits go way beyond the mat. Along the way, I will be referring to some of the ancient texts as well as to many of the incredible scholars, teachers, therapists, practitioners, academics and scientists whose research and experience further enrich and expand my own knowledge and understanding of yoga, which dates back thirty years. In fact, I started yoga and first embarked on my own therapy at about the same time. I can see now that I was clearly seeking any method available to ease my pain – I didn't care how, I just wanted it to stop. What I couldn't see then was how both approaches would slowly and gently help me to rewire the old, entrenched ways of being and doing that were contributing to that unhappiness. I didn't know there was another way to be; I thought that was just my personality, that was just how the world worked. Together, yoga and psychotherapy, each in its own miraculous way, helped bring to consciousness the realisation that I had choices, that I didn't have to do things the way I had always done them, that emotion didn't have to be something to be feared, that people weren't necessarily relating to me in the ways I imagined they were. But it was really only years later, when I embarked on my psychotherapy training and deepened my yoga enquiry further, that I fully understood the similarities between the two. I would read authors (such as Candace Pert, Bessel van der Kolk, Babette Rothschild, Stephen Cope, John Chitty, Pat Ogden, Dan Siegel and so many more) who were writing about embodied emotions and mind–body unity in ways that were both yogic and psychotherapeutic and I would find myself confused as to whether I had originally picked up the book as research for my psychotherapy course or my yoga course, such was the overlap.

But this is not only my story. Stories from the Fierce Calm contributors who have found yoga to be their guide, saviour even, through the darker times in their lives are dotted throughout this book. Alongside their brave tales I offer thoughts from my dual perspective of yoga teacher and psychotherapist. Thoughts as to how and why yoga can have such powerful effects and how that might mirror the psychotherapeutic journey.

I have divided the chapters into some of the most common issues modern life has us coping with – anxiety, insecurity, reactivity, overwhelm and so on. In each chapter I will explore how those conditions might have come about and some of the ways in which

Introduction

they manifest. I will then talk a little about how I might work with them, both as a psychotherapist and as a yoga teacher, examining the parallels between these two supposedly so different yet actually so similar disciplines. And then I will offer some suggestions as to which yoga practices, postures or theories might be useful in working with that particular condition or tendency.

The issues I have identified in each chapter are by no means exhaustive and do not generally exist in isolation. None of us ever fits neatly into only one heading; we are all too complex for such easy categorisation. And similarly, one yoga posture can't ever 'cure' such multi-layered issues, especially when taken out of context. So I may suggest a posture or a sequence or a type of yoga but just because I mention a particular thing doesn't mean it will 'work' for you, nor will it work alone, nor outside the context of a regular yoga practice. It is called a practice for a reason, because it is in the repetition and deepening ongoing enquiry that yoga can affect us. Just as our issues, concerns or preoccupations tend to be multi-faceted – anxiety often goes alongside depression, trauma with addiction, lack of self-care with overly caretaking others and so on – so too is the route to healing. No one yoga posture will do everything, it's the combination and the attitude with which one practises them that effectuates transformation.

In the words of naturalist and author John Muir (1838–1914):

When we try to pick out anything by itself, we find it hitched to everything else in the universe.[1]

So true. And just as we too are a whole, interconnected system of mind, body, thoughts, emotions, bones, muscles, organs, identities, so is yoga a holistic practice. I hope this book will reflect that.

Please bear in mind that some postures, techniques or ideas from psychotherapy or any story or experience you read about here may not resonate with you. Some parts may only make sense after you have investigated and practised yoga more, or some may never do so. Use this book, and the ideas within, in whatever way works for you, knowing that I will be alongside you on that journey, hopefully providing a bit of gentle encouragement from the mat next to yours.

You may have some questions now, let me answer them here.

What is yoga, what is psychotherapy and what do they have to do with each other?

Good questions.

Let's start with yoga, and with what it is not. It is not a way of punishing your body into submission or trying to make it look a certain way. It has nothing to do with appearance or image at all. Yoga is about how it feels on the inside and about developing a relationship with yourself.

What yoga is, too, is a framework for living. Originally it was largely concerned with breath, meditation, chanting, ethics and philosophy, but that has evolved to include a moving practice of physical postures. A practice including all of this can contribute to psychological growth.

I'd like to emphasise the word 'practice' here because I'm not talking about something you do once, or once in a while, but something that you regularly engage with and which is integral to how you live your life.

We will look at many of the elements, including, of course, the postures themselves (in Sanskrit, *asanas*), as well as ways of sequencing them, plus the attitude, pace and energetic focus you bring to them. Postures do not exist in a vacuum.

Introduction

Because yoga emerged from the East many millennia ago, I like to use the original Sanskrit words as much as possible. It reminds me that by practising yoga I am connecting to something deeper, richer, more spiritual even, than just a series of exercises. Sanskrit reminds me that I am a Westerner learning from an Eastern, venerable, very ancient tradition that has much to teach me. I never want to forget who made it possible, and from whom I am imbibing this great culture that is not my own. I want to acknowledge my gratitude for the generosity with which this hard-won knowledge has been shared throughout the ages and across the globe, and which I, and the others sharing their stories, are honoured to play a tiny, tiny part in disseminating further.

So what about psychotherapy, then?

Broadly, psychotherapy is a process in which client and therapist together explore what in the client's history has shaped them to become the person they are, by examining their past, present and future, and – if the client has a belief system or philosophy – possibly the next life as well. This developing self-knowledge brings in its wake more options, including the option to change the behaviours and habits that no longer serve them.

As with my definition of yoga, this is simplified. In neither case have I really even touched the sides of such powerful and life-changing processes, but we are at the start of our journey together, and much more about both disciplines will emerge over the course of this book.

Why do I put the two together?

For oh so many reasons, starting with the fact that both offer us the opportunity to experience ourselves in new ways; ways that can help us better bear the unbearable, while discovering more joy in the pleasurable.

Both are holistic, with psychotherapy becoming more so in recent years as the profession realises just how essential it is to be more than simply a 'talking cure'. Most therapists now keep the body, the emotions and the relationship between themself and their client very much in mind. More broadly, psychotherapy is opening up to the influence of disciplines such as neuroscience, neurobiology, psychosomatics and psychoneuroimmunology that recognise and investigate the inseparability of mind and body. We now understand the interconnectedness and mutual influence of our thoughts, behaviours and emotions with our nervous, endocrine, respiratory and immune systems. These are connections the yogis have long explored via their practice, and which science is now able to prove more measurably.

Yoga and psychotherapy both look behind the surface symptom to the deeper causes of our ills. Both recognise our complexity. Both encourage and aid us to nurture and develop our self-awareness, groundedness, attunement and compassion. Both offer us a way of recognising, acknowledging and, most importantly, being with those aspects of ourselves which we find hardest to bear, while freeing us from old, unhelpful and limiting patterns. Both can help us maximise our potential to live a better, more personally satisfying life.

Much of this relates to what is going on internally in the relationship between our body and mind. But both yoga and therapy also help us connect and relate better externally too, improving our relationships with others individually and collectively.

Do I need both?

Possibly, yes. I am not suggesting that yoga is a replacement for psychotherapy. Each will hugely enhance the other if practised

Introduction

together, but some of the issues we look at in this book may need professional clinical help as well; in these cases yoga should be thought of as a valuable adjunct to psychotherapy.

What both yoga and psychotherapy ultimately give you are benefits, skills and new ways of experiencing yourself that you can take away and use beyond the mat and outside the therapy room. These will endure because you will have absorbed them not only in your mind or your body, but through what is called the 'bodymind'.

This word may sound 'out there'; but it is actually a fairly common term in psychotherapy as well as in yoga, and is really just a handy way to not have to endlessly say, 'When I say body I don't mean the body is separate from the mind, and when I say mind I am not excluding the body, I mean the whole system working together as one.'

One final thought

We are all works in progress. Nothing and no one remains static; we evolve and change, and that is a good thing. Psychotherapy as a profession has also evolved – from the early Freudian discoveries, through years of developments, to the current embracing of neuroscience and other disciplines – each new learning building on and adding to what we already know. Yoga too is always evolving and embracing influences from the varied societies it now serves, without losing touch with its roots.

If we don't adapt, we don't thrive. We don't discard the past, but we don't have to be constrained by it; we can build on it. That is true for us as individuals, it is true in yoga and it is true in psychotherapy. With yoga and psychotherapy as your guides, your own evolution can be supported and nurtured.

Yoga Saved My Life
Ruthie Hanan

I've been in and out of the hospital from age fifteen. I've dealt with chronic illness and had a back brace, so I spent most of my childhood and adolescence assuming that I'm more delicate than others. I had my colon removed, and had a long and painful recovery, physically and mentally.

Throughout, I am positive I would have given up if yoga hadn't found me. It was the first time I'd heard of accepting the state you are in. With painkillers being fed to me at an insane rate, the idea of actually feeling the pain was something new and interesting. If I don't feel this pain, how will I ever move on? This fuels my daily yoga practice: feeling my feelings.

When we shove things down deep, their echo reverberates through our being. Yoga and meditation taught me to feel my feelings as they come. Feel and release them.

This is the process of clearing the mind and finding ourselves under all the layers life creates. Yoga has been here for thousands of years and there's a reason. I'm forever grateful for the process of yoga, the syncing of mind and body.

The longest journey is the journey inward.
                                          Dag Hammarskjold

CHAPTER ONE

Stressed Out

Yoga Saved My Life
Helen Bashford

I learned early on in my childhood to rely on no one and to zone out when something kicked off.

I left home with a stubborn determination to prove my worth. I studied psychology and had a career in mental health but in hindsight this perpetuated old patterns. I often worked with violent people and it's only now I realise I spent most of my twenties living in a permanent state of high alert. My career helped me understand those around me, but it never taught me anything about me. I started yoga at eighteen and my love for it has come less from what I learn on the mat and more from what I learn off it. Studying the science of yoga has taught me everything about me. I understand how my childhood shaped my brain and nervous system. I understand why I can't tolerate raised voices, being ignored, belittled or in the spotlight and see how my negative reactions affect my relationships. Yoga has given me the confidence to remove toxic people from my life.

It has taught me how to read my body. I feel stress signals from my nervous system before my mind even registers there's a problem, giving me more control over my reactions.

Yoga has saved my sanity.

Let's start our yogic exploration with something that most of us will recognise all too well. Stress. Barely any of us are immune. The hectic, busy, technology-heavy and increasingly also frightening and uncertain times we live in have made it pervasive across practically all cultures and societies. Whatever our own particular circumstances, most of us spend most of our time feeling like we are nowhere near on top of all the things that we should be on top of. This has mental, emotional and physical repercussions: an irritability of mood alongside irritating aching in our joints; a racing heartbeat accompanying racing thought patterns; a lack of mental concentration attending our lack of physical energy; not to mention leaking orifices – sweat from our bodies, tears from our eyes.

I have chosen to start our yogic and therapeutic exploration here not only because stress is such a common problem that we can all easily relate to it, but also precisely because it shows how closely those mental, physical and emotional states are aligned, as Helen's story above describes so well.

Stress can feel like a permanent state of affairs. But initially it starts as a response to an external trigger – a work deadline or a family argument, for instance – and in an ideal world (ha!) should dissipate once the issue has been sorted. When left unresolved, however – like Helen's problems – continued stress can lead to long-term problems.

Physically, that might include heart attacks or a stroke, or compromised immune, digestive and respiratory systems.

Cognitively, it can lead to disorganised thinking, outbursts of rage and frustration, poor choices and so much more.

Emotionally, it plays havoc, often leading to anxiety, depression or both.

Stress and the Autonomic Nervous System

Nothing illuminates the holistic nature of our bodymind like the autonomic nervous system. It intricately connects, affects and reflects the state of both body and mind. As Helen discovered, a healthy nervous system allows us to regulate our stress levels. And it responds beautifully to yoga. Our yoga practice therefore gives us the tools to manipulate (in the nicest possible way) our physiological and emotional states.

Page 22 goes into greater detail about the autonomic nervous system, but broadly, it tells us whether people, places and things feel safe or dangerous; allows us to engage with others; and it manages our energy levels – either energetic alertness or calm clarity, both of which we need at different times of the day, and in different circumstances. However, if you have experienced stress – and quite frankly, who hasn't – then you will have felt in a very real way the physical, mental and emotional upheaval that arises when the nervous system unleashes chemical messengers working overtime to relay the news, across body and mind, that 'all is not well'. Our ability to connect with others and benefit from their support is affected, which in itself affects stress levels if compromised. This can lead the nervous system to lean too heavily on what is called its sympathetic half and overly energise us so we become hyper-stimulated or stressed; or it veers too heavily towards the other, parasympathetic, half, which can numb us to the point of shutting us down and taking away motivation or the ability to change.

Stress and Psychotherapy

Many of the clients arriving in my consulting room have been brought there by the overwhelm of a stressful situation, or an ongoing stressful life. They often tell me long, convoluted stories about all the ins and outs of the problem. They – and I, if I am not careful – can get bogged down in the sheer volume of information, bamboozled by every last little detail. But the detail is rarely the point; what has to be dealt with first is the effect of the overwhelm, because no problem is ever solved from a state of agitation.

Even though many think of therapy as a 'talking cure', this is a good example of how the verbal is not always what is important – it is the whole bodymind that has to be attended to, just as it is in yoga. So, as a therapist hearing the client's story of stress for the first time, I need to 'tune out' the *content* and instead 'tune in' to the *tone* in which it is being conveyed. I need to simplify the *details* in favour of the *emotion* behind it, to take the heat out of it.

I also need to try to help my client turn the focus away from the outside world with all its problems, and turn it towards their internal state.

We all need to remember we are human beings, not human doings. We need to bring the focus back to us, make it less about others. Often I try to encourage a client to stop talking about themselves as 'you' and say 'I' instead. For instance, clients will often say something like: 'when it's all you're thinking about, and you're so busy all the time you can't switch off...' Compare the feeling that evokes to 'when it's all *I'm* thinking about, and *I'm* so busy all the time *I* can't switch off...' If we can focus on ourselves there is a qualitatively different shift in perspective.

Part of what helps this turning inwards and back towards a calmer state is the feeling of being 'held' by a reliable other, your psychotherapist, with whom you feel safe and have a relationship of trust.

Stressed Out

Stress and Yoga

Outside the therapy room, yoga can teach you how to find self-regulation; how to turn inwards safely, gain a trusting relationship with yourself, and use those tools to help calm and ground you. As Helen says, 'I feel stress signals from my nervous system before my mind even registers there's a problem, giving me more control over my reactions.' Learning to notice your own physical cues to your stress levels will similarly give you a greater feeling of control, and this is another skill that yoga can help you develop over time.

If stress is an 'accelerator' that we step on in our full-throttle bid to get the job/confrontation/problem 'sorted', what we need to balance it out is a yoga practice that acts as the 'brake' and helps us introduce a bit of calm.

And we know that yoga can do this. Yogis have known for years that yoga helps to balance the autonomic nervous system and makes us feel better all round as a result. And now science is catching up and validating yogis' experiential accounts. People working in all different areas of science are doing this – neuroscientists, endocrinologists, academics – and they are all discovering the same, *measurable* thing – yoga reduces stress.[2] It has been seen to change the brain itself, allowing new neural pathways to grow, strengthening the communication between those pathways, increasing beneficial hormone production and distribution, decreasing the size of the amygdala (the brain's fire alarm) and making it less reactive and having a valuable effect on our heart-rate variability – one of the most reliable measures of how responsive we are to stress.

So what sort of yoga practice is going to best help do this?

The first thing to say is that any general, well-balanced yoga practice can reduce stress. The clue lies in the word 'balanced' – I mean here a practice that gives equal attention to all aspects of the nervous system. One which alternates activity with rest, challenge with kindness, the front of the body with the back, the left with the right and so on. This will not only even out the internal and external body physically, but will simultaneously bring a state of balance, of equanimity, to the mind. The mind follows the body, which follows the mind, in a virtuous circle. Calm one and you calm the other; they are not actually separate.

However, if you are very stressed and you already know that you need serenity and composure far more than you need activation, then you can be more directive about it. The suggestions below show how you can tailor your yoga to focus specifically on quietening the energising, sympathetic element of the nervous system while promoting the soothing parasympathetic, thus gently nudging yourself into a calmer state. This works both ways, incidentally, and we will look at the flip side of this – kick-starting a sluggish nervous system – in the depression chapter (Chapter 3).

- **A slower practice**

This first suggestion is quite simple really: slow down your movements. Take longer to do each posture and slow the transitions between them.

Well, I say it's simple but I know that in reality, slowing down can be hard. So do it gradually. If you are very stressed – your mind whirring and your body jittery – then you are unlikely to be able go straight into a slower practice as you will be too wired. You may need to start off with some active movements and then gradually slow down, minute by minute. Like easing your foot slowly down onto the brake rather than slamming into a jarring emergency stop. You may even want to start a session by shaking out different parts of the body in turn, or dancing, to dissipate built-up energy.

Something that may help you to move at a less frantic pace is to slow your breathing. There will be more about breathing later in the book as it is so fundamental to yoga. For now, though, just know that your movements should always be led by your breath (by which I mean, for example, start to breathe in and allow that feeling of lifting to initiate, for instance, a corresponding raising of your arms). Reducing your speed may help this connection become more evident and also more natural.

You may start to notice that when stressed you tend to breathe more shallowly, using only the top part of your lungs. This is a natural response, but one which stresses the body, leaving it feeling as though it is not being properly 'fed' with the oxygen it so desperately needs. It also stresses the brain because a lack of oxygen sends the message that you are in danger and can eventually provoke a fight-or-flight response.

A slower practice provides the time and space to breathe from the abdomen. This mimics what you do naturally when relaxed, so sends the message to your brain that you are safe.

Changes in breath can change the biochemistry of the brain.[3] Whatever version of yoga you are working with, your breathing should always be a fundamental starting point.

- **Lengthen the exhale**

An inhalation invigorates the sympathetic (activating) nervous system, inflating and expanding the body and readying it for action. An exhalation, on the other hand, encourages the parasympathetic (calming) nervous system to kick in as you expel the air, allowing your body to gently release and soften as it 'deflates', knowing its work is done.

So while you are slowing down movement and breath, see if you can also slightly extend the length of your exhalation in relation to your inhalation.

Certain postures naturally encourage a longer, deeper exhalation, so choose wisely, and see my next suggestion.

- **Forward bends**

We've just seen that exhaling helps nudge us further towards parasympathetic activation. Forward bends happen most easily on an exhalation so it's a natural pairing – as we expel air, our bodies take up less space, contracting, emptying and folding in on themselves, taking us naturally into a forward bend. Our awareness moves inwards, we soften, we release; the physical movement, as we have seen, affects us physiologically and emotionally.

We can tend to forget or disregard the back of the body, and in a way it is more 'private' than the front, orienting away from the world and other people. Bending forwards allows the outward-facing front of the body to take a break, instead stretching and taking the focus towards the back. The inhalation is compromised – actually a good thing in this context as it forces the breath to find other space to move into, which it does by reaching deeper into the often more neglected back of the lungs, bringing awareness and life to the spine and back of the body. Restful *balasana*, child's pose, is particularly good for this.

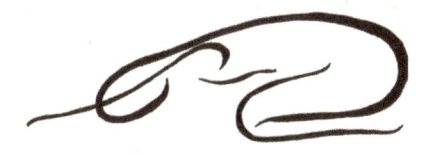

Balasana

Forward bending also takes us closer to the floor so we get a better sense of grounding and anchoring, which can be a good tether if the stress has had us feeling we are floating somewhere above the ground in a flurry of activity. Turning the focus away from the outside world in this way encourages introspection and, symbolically, the sense of yielding inwards and downwards can engender feelings of release into something greater – a return to the trusted solidity of the Earth, which is always there to catch us. This pose brings the heart higher than the head, symbolising how it is the heart that should really be guiding us.

A deep forward fold that compresses the internal organs can also help replenish the kidneys. The kidneys are significant due to their proximity and intimate connection to the adrenal glands, which release stress hormones and so become overworked if we are frequently or chronically stressed. The replenishment of a deep forward fold can be calming and restorative to them. Kidneys, when healthy, also remove excess waste, acting as a filter system, and releasing hormones that regulate blood pressure to help reduce stress further.

The Autonomic Nervous System

The autonomic nervous system (ANS) manages our automatic functions such as blood pressure, heart rate, digestion, body temperature and so on. It affects our energy, our overall health and our ability to regulate our responses and even mediates how much we feel able to either engage with, or need to withdraw from, the world and other people, acting as our inner alarm system, scanning the environment for cues of safety or danger and responding accordingly.

Traditionally we've understood the ANS as a binary system – either energised or calm – but more recent research now tells us that it in fact operates in three modes, better described as calm connection, mobilisation or immobilisation.

We will look more in later chapters at what happens when the ANS detects danger – this is when immobilisation is more likely to come into play – but for now let's look at how it functions when we feel safe, healthy and socially engaged. Such a state is characterised by a nervous system which can move fluidly from one mode to another. This means that our sympathetic nervous system speeds up our breathing and heart rate, energising us and helping us get up and out, enabling us to be productive, creative and extroverted. It is our 'accelerator', counterbalanced by our 'brake', the parasympathetic nervous system, which contrastingly slows down our breathing and heart rate, calming us and enabling us to be more introverted and do things that need a bit of peace and quiet, like sleep and digesting food. Here is also the home of our vagus nerve, which, when 'toned' means our social engagement system functions optimally, allowing us to connect with others to further aid the fluid pendulation between states.

Modern life tends to interrupt this gentle and harmonious swing to and fro, however. Our body's natural tendency to seek equanimity and balance can take a bit of a knocking by daily stresses, meaning one mode gets overactivated at the expense of the other. The result is that we often override our body's natural attempts to balance and harmonise by using caffeine, sugar or workaholism to artificially keep us in sympathetic-dominant mode, constantly on the go, beyond the point where we can naturally calm down. We then turn to other types of behaviours – drugs or alcohol for instance – to help push us back into the parasympathetic mode that we've spent all day overriding.

Yoga can help us to rediscover a more natural balance by allowing the body to gently find its way back into homeostasis. And by regulating ourselves physically, our minds and emotions too can fluidly alternate from energised to calm, as needed. The emotional regulation comes hand in hand with the physical – when we are physiologically more balanced, we are more emotionally balanced as well, and vice versa.

Neither mode of the nervous system is either good or bad. We need a bit more of each at different times, depending on situation, environment and time of day. We need the transitions between them to be smooth, so we can sway effortlessly from one to the other according to the

> demands of the moment. The problems only emerge when we get stuck longer than necessary in one mode, at the expense of the other.
> Yoga can help unstick us.

We should not pretend to understand the world only by the intellect; we apprehend it just as much by feeling. Therefore, judgment of the intellect is, at best, only the half of truth, and must, if it be honest, also come to an understanding of its inadequacy.

Carl Jung

CHAPTER TWO

Anxiety Rules

Yoga Saved My Life
Danni Pomplun

Before yoga there was drinking, drugs, anxiety, depression – I succumbed to all of it. Met with an ultimatum from my roommate, it was either do something constructive and restorative with myself, or move out.

Yoga and meditation entered my life because I didn't have a choice. I didn't go to classes and keep up with the practice because I wanted to; I did it because I HAD to. On my own terms, I let yoga into my life after noticing the physical, mental and emotional changes from within.

Yoga never cared that I was hungover from the night before. It never judged me for my past. It held me up with every pose. It has been a practice that is there for me whenever I need, be it in times of happiness, injury, exhaustion, non-stop tears… it's been there.

This practice we do, we don't do alone. We come to our mats and dedicate the time for ourselves to better ourselves, which betters the people we interact with.

Asana after asana, breath by breath, we foster a community of mutual love and respect from which we grow, nurture and support each other. And that's what I love about this practice.

When stress becomes chronic it can lead to anxiety. Anxiety strikes many of us from time to time, while others among us suffer it almost constantly to the point where it rules our lives, often feeling pressure to 'do it all'.

While stress is generally triggered by an external event or threat that can be tackled, and so (in theory) obviating the need for the stress, anxiety tends to be more of an internal feeling of apprehension or dread that often has no obvious cause and persists even when the initial concern has passed.

Whether anxiety is a constant companion or an infrequent visitor, yoga is a good antidote, as numerous studies have found.[4] Many of us don't need science to tell us this; we have found that yoga can help us figure out how to work with anxiety and sit with discomfort. The yoga mat can become a safe place to do that.

Why and How Does Yoga Help with Anxiety?

Anxiety is quite a general term and it affects different people in different ways; but, like stress, it is often characterised by racing, uncontrollable thoughts speeding towards the worst possible conclusions, sometimes accompanied by sweating and a feeling that your heart is beating too quickly. It can be frightening and exhausting as those intrusive thoughts go round and round, spiralling through an ever-worsening litany of worries, with each worry kick-starting the next. While we tend to think of anxiety as predominantly a 'thinking' thing, the body too (remember they are never really separate) is also in a constant of state of high alert: tight, tense, gripped, primed for danger and unable to let go what it feels as a need for vigilance.

Anxiety Rules

Yoga can interrupt that cycle.

One of the earliest known yoga texts, the *Yoga Sutras*, says that the purpose of yoga is to 'still the fluctuations of the mind' (in Sanskrit, *citta vrtti nirodhah*). If ever there were a perfect summary of what a person with anxiety needs, it is this. So how does yoga go about stilling the fluctuations of that oh-so-disobedient mind?

Well, there are a few ways, but a lot of it comes down to focus and the concentration needed to get your body into – and to stay in – certain positions or shapes. This both stops the mind wandering elsewhere, and also keeps your attention rooted in the physical as opposed to mental oscillations.

Any yoga practice will encourage you to constantly bring your mind back to what you are doing in the moment and so promote concentration. However, there are a couple of types of postures that I would single out.

• Balancing postures

I love how symbolic the balancing postures are in paving the way towards emotional balance, while also strengthening and fortifying our ability to literally balance.

There are so many opposites in our lives, so many things competing to pull us in different directions, it's no wonder our brains can't still themselves, can't remain focused on just the task in hand. But when the task in hand is staying upright on one leg, and the price for not doing so is falling flat on your face, the incentive to concentrate is pretty compelling. The physical practice of balancing works simultaneously on mental and emotional levels, the stillness of body and breath promoting mental clarity. And we now know, from neuroscientific research, that on a very concrete level, balancing postures are even able to actually rewire the brain, creating new neural pathways.[5]

Next time you do a balancing posture pay attention to what your mind is doing. Take *vrksasana*, tree pose, one of the most common balances. Notice what happens when you begin. If you are very wobbly, that might be an indicator that your mind is not on an even keel. Not only does what we do with the body affect the mind, but the opposite is also true; if the mind is scattered and jumpy, the body will be too. Straight away you can see your ability, or not, to balance, as a sign that you are a bit all over the place. Quite literally.

Two things are going to help you alleviate the wobbliness.

- First, fix your gaze on one point in the middle distance and keep it there. Stilling the eyes, not allowing them to dart about, is the first indicator to your mind and body that you need to be still now. By focusing the eyes, we simultaneously start to focus the mind away from extraneous thoughts, and also the body, which starts to quiet itself. It all works in tandem.
- Secondly, try to bring your inner focus down from the mind into the body, to where it really matters right now if you are to stay standing. Your stability will come, in large part, from the one foot that is still on the floor. So, bring your awareness down into the sole of the foot. Picture its broadness. Feel into the base of the big toe, then the base of the little toe, the inner edge of the heel, the outer edge of the heel. Notice how by bringing your attention to ever smaller parts of the body, thinking about how supported you are, and by focusing on broadening your base, your mind has stopped worrying about the state of the economy or whether you said a stupid thing in today's meeting and is instead completely absorbed in the moment. The fluctuations of your mind have stilled. Maybe only for a few

brief moments – but that is a few more moments of respite than you had before you did it. And just as your mind has stopped jumping about all over the place, you may find that your body has quieted as well.

With my psychotherapist hat in place, I can see that this parallels how I might work with an anxious client. What the balancing posture helps us do physically – interrupt frantic thinking and bring the awareness into the body – is what a therapist sometimes needs to help a client do verbally. With an anxious client I might spend a lot of time asking them to engage with the feeling, not the thought. I might need to repeatedly ask them to stop telling me what they think and instead start telling me how they feel; encourage them to spend less time in their thoughts and more time in their feelings.

Why?

Well, anxiety can be a defence against feelings that we fear may overwhelm us, flooding us with more than we can bear. We reside more and more insistently in our brains, believing (wrongly) that we can think our way through the problem, as opposed to using sensations and feelings to guide us in another way. We may feel cut off from our feelings to the extent that we cannot even recognise things like hunger or fear or pain because we are so determined to override annoyances like that by sheer force of will. We resolutely refuse to acknowledge that our bodies have anything to offer.

We all have defences that we use to shield ourselves from frightening emotions – this one, this going up into the head, is called intellectualising. As a therapist, my job in these instances is to help an anxious person understand that their emotional intelligence is just as important as their intellectual intelligence and so help them get more into their feelings safely and understand why feelings might hold such terror.

Yoga helps you connect with your feelings safely, giving you another way of experiencing your body. A certain posture might help you contact an unexpected feeling in a safer and previously unexplored way, and thus open a door into deeper exploration with your therapist. Conversely, it may also lead you to a place where you don't feel safe – and that might be something that you can then take to your therapist so that together you can work on understanding why this might be so.

Your yoga practice can open a door into a new, more trusting way of experiencing what it feels like to have a place that never changes and never judges.

Therapy and yoga, when we are working with anxiety, both encourage us to focus on the support we can get from our bodies if we can loosen the grip on our minds. And they can both help us harness our thoughts more productively so as not to drown in anxious feelings.

- **Challenging postures**

My second suggestion is to challenge yourself occasionally with a new or complicated posture. What this means to you will, of course, depend on your experience and your own tendencies, so don't take my suggestions as instructions. But just as an example, a posture with many things going on at once, like revolved half-moon (*parivrtta ardha chandrasana* in Sanskrit) – where not only are you balancing but you are also twisting and side bending all within one posture – will give you so many different aspects to focus on at once that you cannot fail but be completely absorbed.

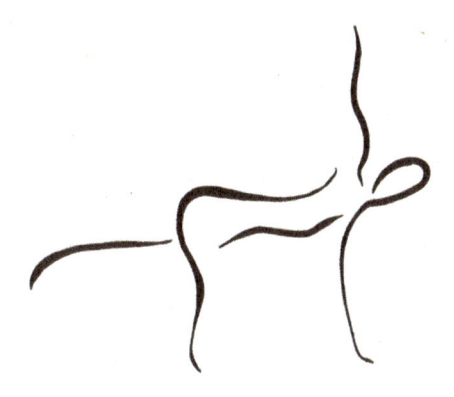

Parivrtta Ardha Chandrasana

Another benefit of this is that it will put the body under such (beneficial) physical stress that, possibly counterintuitively, when you learn that with better breathing and focus you can withstand this, when you learn that it passes, then you are training your nervous system to understand that the body's physiological response doesn't have to just react but can relax, even during times of stress.

Anxiety, Stress and the Endocrine System

The three major stress hormones are adrenaline, cortisol and norepinephrine. They are released when the bodymind becomes alerted to threat. This can take the form of an advancing tiger, a looming deadline or the suspicion that your spouse might be having an affair. That is to say it can be concrete, abstract or even imaginary. The bodymind can't necessarily always tell the difference, so it will react in a similar way no matter how large, small, real or imagined the threat.

And the way it reacts is primarily physiological; there is a very real sequence of events going on inside our bodies' cells. This is why simply telling ourselves not to be silly, or to calm down, is not always helpful.

When faced with a threat the hypothalamus (in the brain) alerts the pituitary gland, which, in turn, sends its chemical messages to the adrenal glands – in the body – telling them to release those stress hormones. See again how we cannot separate body and brain? The two have different roles but are working in conjunction.

Those stress hormones mobilise other systems, such as the respiratory and the cardiovascular, and soon our entire network is flooded with these shouty little doom-mongers and is jumping to their tune, the tune of panic and stress. This is a very useful response in the moment of danger, but not always so useful if they carry on shouting beyond the time when action is actually needed. The nervous system is, of course, responding as well. It will either activate the sympathetic nervous system to ready us for fight or flight by increasing our heart, blood pressure and respiration rates, mobilising our muscles and altering our body temperature, or it will activate the immobilisation part of our parasympathetic nervous system in order to shut us down completely.

It is possible, however, to learn to manage and quiet this physiological message – yoga and therapy being two of the most effective ways.

Why is it important to learn ways of managing our responses? Well, it makes life more comfortable for a start. But it also stops things from getting worse, which can easily happen as a vicious circle gets under way: the more stress that is triggered, the more sensitive all those systems become to it, and the easier it is to trigger it, so it happens more and more often, and the harder it becomes to shut it off. And the long-term effects can be dangerous in ways that affect other systems in the body including the immune, digestive and reproductive systems. We can become more prone to heart attack, stroke, insomnia, premature ageing; the neural networks in the brain can get rewired, leading to moodiness, loneliness, addictions, poor concentration and memory, negativity, poor judgement, and more prone to anxiety and depression. It's a gloomy list, all right. But fear not, yoga is going to help.

A purely disembodied human emotion is a non-entity.
William James, 1884

CHAPTER THREE

When Depression Strikes

Yoga Saved My Life
Jessica Wilson-Thille

I suffered from depression throughout my childhood, and it became particularly vicious in high school.

I was put on antidepressants, for which I am actually very grateful; I had no other way of addressing my depression – and they honestly did help. In 1999, I left for college, where I enrolled in yoga as an extra-curricular.

The mindfulness meditation and breathwork, combined with the physical asana, began to open my eyes to a different way of viewing my mind.

I still remember the day I threw my meds away and said, 'I can face this differently'.

I have now been eighteen years meds-free. Has it been hard? Yes. Were there times when I felt like I had no control and maybe needed meds again? Hell, yes!

Did my depression go away? No. But yoga has given me the tools to see my mind differently, to accept and love my dark side, and recognise that I am complete, whole and unbroken just as I am.

When Depression Strikes

Depression is pervasive in our society and can be debilitating, causing life to feel like a miserable struggle, everything in it hopeless and grey. At its worst, it can lead to suicidal thoughts and tragically sometimes actions, can bring other symptoms in its wake – including heart disease or stroke – and can make us old before our time.

There are as many theories as to what causes depression, as there are to what cures it. It is variously thought to be anger turned inwards; a lack of meaning or purpose; a paucity of connection to others; or having no agency over your own life. Some believe it is more physical in origin and due to a chemical imbalance in the brain, inflammation, or because of genetics.

Whatever the cause, it is generally characterised physically and emotionally by a shutting down, a going inwards, a lack of energy or enthusiasm or motivation. It is something I have suffered with all my life, so I feel very familiar with the deadening effects it can bring, the feelings of pointlessness and inertia. I have found it useful to understand what is going on for me on both emotional and physical levels when this happens. It helps stop me descending into self-blame and self-loathing and prevents me from piling on a layer of disgust about the fact that I have no reason to feel like this when I am so lucky and privileged in so many ways. That is not a helpful cognitive filter through which to further beat yourself up when so much pain is already going on.

Physiologically, depression can often involve a nervous system imbalance. We have seen with stress and anxiety what can happen when the sympathetic nervous system dominates, trapping us in accelerator mode – overly hyped up and wired – and we've looked at how yoga can be used to calm that down and promote a move towards the calming influence of the parasympathetic nervous system.

Depression, however, is more often characterised by the opposite problem – we feel heavy, deadened, lethargic and cannot find any energy, enthusiasm or motivation. Here we can use yoga to wake and rouse ourselves.

This lack of energy that we often find in depression can mean that it is your parasympathetic nervous system that is dominating. There is too much pressure on the brake, not enough on the accelerator.

Yoga has helped me massively with my depression, and it can help you too. It can work directly on your depressed nervous system and encourage you and your body to open up more towards the outside world, be less shut down, less inward looking. Because of the intimate connection between body and mind this physical opening up and energising can lead to an emotional opening up and a feeling of greater hopefulness as well. Jessica describes being opened up to a different way of viewing her mind, of facing things differently. You too can start to see – as I have also learned to do – that you do have agency, you can affect your own story, you can make changes, however small, that will slowly act as footholds to guide you up and out of that well of misery.

These are exactly the same things I would incorporate in my work with a depressed client in my therapy room. Alongside trying to understand what has brought them so low, I'd be thinking about finding ways to help them open up more to the outside world and counteract the deadening feeling that accompanies depression. And that's the same path a yoga practice can take. Yoga can't necessarily help you understand and get to the bottom of the experiences that brought you to be being depressed in the first place, but it can alleviate and counteract your symptoms to the point of giving you enough oomph and motivation to be able to explore it more within therapy. And it can help manage the depression neurobiologically, and significantly improve your quality of life.

When Depression Strikes

You can think of yoga as a tool of empowerment rather than necessarily an attempt to solve. And that is very useful, as chances are that someone who is depressed will be sick to death of being told how to solve the problem. They don't want more solutions, they want to learn how to feel differently.

This is particularly relevant when as a therapist I look at how closely the depressed person's mood is reflected in their very being. I can see body language and posture that show a mood that is lethargic, unmotivated, sunken. A person with depression is often slightly folded in on themselves, rounded forwards, as though they are using their back as a shield – like a tortoise or crab does, curling in as a natural response to danger, to protect their vulnerable inner organs and softer parts. Sadly this physical posture, while it might feel comforting and protective, is actually feeding back the depressing messaging, making the problem worse.

So, how can you tailor your yoga practice to interrupt this negative circle of depression?

- **Backbends**

We have seen how forward bends, on both anatomical and metaphorical levels, help gently alleviate stress. Backbends, working in the same way but in the opposite direction, can do the same for depression.

A backbend can gently counteract the depressed person's hunched, defensive posture by stretching and lengthening the front of the body, encouraging the tender, softer side to come out of hiding, open towards the light of day and engage with the outside world.

We saw how forward bends encourage a lengthening of the exhalation and activate the parasympathetic nervous system. Contrastingly, backbends open the front of the body to promote a longer inhalation, which invigorates the sympathetic nervous system which energises and wakes us. We can kick-start re-engagement and vitality, unleashing a natural internal 'caffeine supply' and aiding our opening to the world to bring us back to life.

Backbends lengthen the neck and lift the head, encouraging us to face up and out, taking us away from introspection and instead asking us to reach towards the sky with all its potential and possibility. This lifting and lengthening is a great antidote to the droopy roundedness we feel when depressed, that posture which represents the feeling that we are carrying the weight of the world on our shoulders. Backbends are also fantastic, over time, for strengthening the shoulder girdle and its associated muscles. As well as making us physically stronger, this gives us symbolic fortitude, helping us feel we can now shoulder that burden more effectively, while the increasingly stronger back muscles similarly provide a sense of being able to combat the downward pull of depression.

As the back strengthens, the chest opens. Depression can often involve the opposite problem to stress, which can make us lose touch with our inner world; a depressed person tends to feel too inward looking, too separate, isolated and alone, so opening the chest and bringing the attention to the outward-facing front of the body reminds us there is an outside world towards which we can reach.

The opening engendered will release emotions, however. Part of the folding inwards of depression is to protect and hide from deep feelings. We roll into a ball or a foetal position when feeling most attacked. One of the most tender places we are armouring in this way is the heart. By exposing ourselves, by opening the body like this, especially the area around the heart, some of those bottled-up emotions will be released and can find expression. Emotions, like so many things, are generally better out than in. Leading with the heart like this can symbolically teach us to trust our hearts and make decisions from there, not from our heads.

When Depression Strikes

Exposing yourself takes bravery. Yet realising you have survived this exposure builds courage. This reflects one of the benefits of therapy as well – a realisation that connection with your therapist and with more vulnerable parts of yourself shows you that openness can be met with empathy, and can bring rewards. This resulting trust helps you connect to others outside the therapy room and off the yoga mat, enabling you to reap the benefits of external support.

Internally, the abdominal organs get a good stretch, which improves digestion and some of the stagnation that can both fuel, and be exacerbated by, depression's lethargy. We become more open to living our lives more fully and become less shut down – physically and emotionally – to experiences and to other people.

Many backbends invert us, or at least invert our gaze. This change of visual perspective can encourage a new emotional perspective on all that is making us depressed, maybe offering a way out of the hopelessness. Instead of looking at the ground and feeling overwhelmed by the pull of gravity, we are looking up to the open potentiality of the sky, with its limitless possibilities and unrestricted access to fresh air, inspiration, invigoration and optimism.

Backbends tend to be quite challenging; doing them requires a high level of engagement, meaning we have to concentrate more on the breath to help us through, which often stimulates the sympathetic nervous system. Meeting challenges can also show us what we are capable of. I know that in my early days of yoga I absolutely hated backbends. I couldn't foresee a day when this awful combination of contortion and strength wouldn't leave me feeling even more useless than I did already. But that time did come and now I adore backbends. They make me feel alive and strong and they create within me a feeling analogous to a spring day dawning, bursting into flower after a gloomy dead winter.

The curative powers of yoga are as much about an attitude and an approach as they are about the postures themselves. HOW we do our practice is just as important as WHAT we do.

In the chapter on stress I suggested slowing down your practice; now I'm going to talk about not exactly the opposite, but a practice where you keep 'on the go'.

- **Be active**

An active, flowing yoga practice that gets the body moving will work physiologically to get the blood circulating and the oxygen flowing. This all helps to activate the sympathetic nervous system and encourage deeper breathing.

Just as with slowing down your practice, it may be hard to switch gear too rapidly or dramatically. You may need to match your energy to where you are currently in the moment, and recognise that you cannot move much at the start of the practice. So begin gently with simple, possibly supine postures and breathing that matches your current mood. As you gradually move a bit more, and as the body starts to respond, then you can slowly build up to more energetic postures over the course of the session.

- **Do the postures you enjoy**

This suggestion is probably the most important in the whole book and should really be your number-one rule. It is so important: be playful and experimental and try to enjoy your practice.

Quite apart from all the physiological benefits to the body, organs and nervous system, emotionally it may be that by engaging in a sequence or some postures you know you love, you will be able to find joy or at least a sense of pleasure or satisfaction. That may provide a glimpse of a more-alive you, one where sensation and reconnection with yourself and the world can bring pleasure, not just pain. You may find movements and stretches that feel good, and rediscover your sensory pleasure.

Depression can be like a trance of dissociation, an attempt to avoid what hurts us, a numbing of feeling. But not feeling means not living. I know how awful that feels and I know that the answer is for us to bring ourselves back into the world, safely.

We do that by making feeling more obvious, by arousing sensation, by using more expansive movements, by activating a sluggish system. If we have shut down from the bad, we have also shut down from the good, and we need to rediscover the good if we are to help lift depression.

Jessica describes it so well when she realises she can accept and love her darker side, and so feel more 'complete, whole and unbroken' just as she is.

Postures and Sequencing

Yoga incorporates a whole world of things, from physical movement and breathing practices to meditation and a philosophy for life.

But now let's look a bit more closely at the physical side, which consists of a collection of asanas. Commonly translated as 'posture' or 'pose', the word asana is actually more accurately translated as' 'seat'. I think this is important and significant; it can change our thinking about and relationship with the postures if we know that what we are aiming to do within them is find our seat.

We met the *Yoga Sutras* earlier on. Sutra 2.466 tells us '*sthira sukham asanam*', meaning that within each posture we are looking to experience stability and comfort. It's an exhortation often heard at the beginning of a yoga class so as to bring this idea to the forefront of our minds. It has also been translated as 'resolutely abide in a good space'.

The common Western approach to yoga often misses this essential point when it focuses purely on the physical. Even when the postures are challenging, we are aiming to find an easy, steady seat within them. Without this attitude we are just weight training and working up a sweat. With it we start to get in touch with our inner world and learn to create the safe space inside ourselves within which yoga is able to work its magic and save our lives.

But to return to the more prosaic. Each asana has its purpose, strengthening, toning and stretching different parts of the body in turn.

In a way, sequencing works a bit like grammar, with the asanas like words that can be built up into sentences – sequences. And as with grammar, the sequences work best if the asanas are put into a meaningful order.

Just as verbal grammar is made up of nouns, verbs, adjectives and so on, so the asanas are grouped into forward bends, backbends, twists, inversions, standing postures, sitting postures and so on. Some refer to the plane in which the posture is done (standing, sitting, upside down and so on) and some refer to the direction the spine moves in – including extending into a backbend, flexing into a forward bend or rotating into a twist. Ideally a sequence will generally incorporate a varied selection of each, put together in an order that is safe and most beneficial to the spine. The asanas in a sequence can be done statically, or strung together in a moving, dynamic flow called a *vinyasa*.

When Depression Strikes

A classic sequence might proceed something like this:

- It starts with a gentle limbering-up sequence to move the spine in all its six permutations, allowing the body to warm up, the breath to regulate and thoughts to quieten as awareness moves down into the body and away from the head.
- There will often then be a sequence of linked postures called sun salutations (*surya namaskar* in Sanskrit), continuing the theme of moving the spine in all six directions, and warming you further by getting you moving more energetically. This encourages a move to sympathetic nervous system dominance where you are more active and engaged.
- Various asanas will follow, generally focused on building strength and tone. Sometimes there is a theme, often one that allows you to better work certain parts of the anatomy in order to build towards a 'peak' posture, the most challenging of the class, something like a series of backbends leading to *natarajasana* (dancer pose), perhaps, for which you need to be thoroughly warmed up.
- The emphasis will now usually change to more calm-inducing asanas. These will encourage a shift towards the calmness of parasympathetic nervous system dominance and take you towards the slower, more static and relaxing asanas where flexibility rather than strength is more to the fore.
- A class should always end with a period of lying in *savasana* (corpse pose), where the body is allowed to rest, soften and release. It's an essential part of the process as here is where the bodymind is given the time

and space to absorb and be nourished by all the lessons taken on board during the practice.

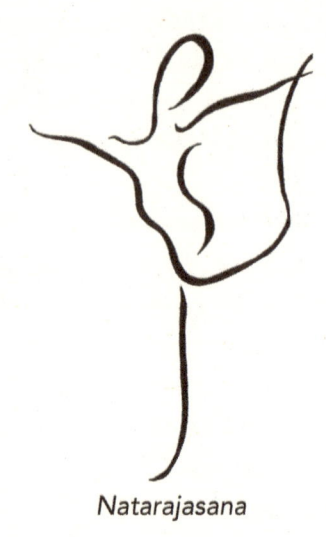

Natarajasana

This is a very broad-brush stroke description of a yoga sequence – they have an infinite variety of permutations – but two things that are pretty much non-negotiable are the warm-up and the concluding *savasana*. The benefits of the warm-up we will look at in more depth later; but *savasana* is equally essential, if less obviously so.

It breaks my heart how often I see people leave a class before *savasana*, seeming to see it as disposable and a waste of time in their efforts to rush on with their day. In fact, it provides crucial absorption of the lessons in balance, of embodying the philosophy that activity needs calm, that challenge needs kindness and that the nervous system needs to recalibrate.

We do not see things as they are. We see them as we are.
                                                          The Talmud

CHAPTER FOUR

Find Some Compassion

Yoga Saved My Life
Dominique Theophilus

I began practising yoga after suffering from anxiety and my body translated it into heart palpitations. I'd feel as if I was about to have a heart attack and it was hard for me to catch my breath. I was unable to sleep.

When I first began, I never truly understood the vastness of yoga: how it would embrace me beyond the physical postures. Yoga created a feeling in me that brought me to tears while at the same time filling me with wholehearted joy afterwards. A balance that was often unexplainable.

Today, yoga and meditation connect my mind, body and spirit. They heal me, allow me to unlearn old patterns and recreate a better version of myself. I love myself more than ever and I love the community I'm a part of.

Yoga is a union, bringing together conversations around race, privilege and other disparities that we often forget about. Centring my work on opening the conversation for communities of colour and traumatic brain injuries, I have discovered humility unlike any other.

Introducing my work to traumatic brain injury clients has been a healing process. They teach and remind me of

> the precious nature of the simplest things in life, like getting dressed in the morning, holding a conversation. They have helped me to understand how to fully embrace being present. As a teacher, I give them the tools of posture and breath, then hold space for them to discover their highest selves. To see these clients evolve and the light in their eyes as they feel a shift in their mental and physical selves cannot be put into words. I'm grateful.

'If I'm not hard on myself, constantly telling myself I can do better, then I will become pathetic and self-pitying.'

This is something I hear far too frequently in my consulting room. The notion that any form of self-compassion is pity, will lead to you being labelled whingey, or a victim, or to the derogatory claim that you are making a fuss about nothing and can't see how lucky you are. Don't you know others have it worse?

Any of these responses sound familiar?

I am willing to bet that they do. Maybe you hear this being said in your mum's voice, or your dad's, perhaps your teacher's. More than likely it's become your own. It could even have turned into the everyday, constant mantra you tell yourself.

Why, as adults, do we consistently tell ourselves the very thing that we used to hate hearing our parents or teachers telling us? It's because our present is informed by our past. A huge amount of psychotherapeutic theory rests on this notion – that our childhood experiences all feed into our present way of being. And many different theorists have come to conceptualise and explain this. One such was John Bowlby. His attachment theory, developed in the 1960s, has become very influential. It postulates that we learn

Find Some Compassion

how to navigate the world via our earliest relationships. It is these that lay down the ground rules for what we can expect from other people, and provide a map for how we should interact with others. As infants our survival is dependent on our caregivers being prepared to continue to care for us. In order to make sure that they do so, we adapt our behaviour to suit them, coming to develop internal rules – or, as he calls them, internal working models – that we follow religiously, even into adulthood when they may no longer be so useful.

So if we grow up in a family environment that prizes self-sufficiency and despises what it might call 'self-pity', then we learn pretty early on to hide those parts of ourselves that might appear to be self-pitying in order to stay in the good books of our caregivers, and keep them onside. This can mean any notion that you deserve compassion gets thrown out, with 'self-pity' becoming a catch-all phrase to dismiss anything, however necessary, that you might need for yourself. In fact, this world view doesn't even have to be articulated; it can be just something we soak up unconsciously as we go along. Children are observant and very good at picking up on non-verbal, nuanced clues as to what is and is not acceptable; what will please our parents and what will anger them. We gradually absorb this information into our very being so that it comes to feel like a part of us, not something we have to consciously think about, just something we naturally do and believe.

Often when I hear a client telling me they don't want to be self-pitying and I ask them whose voice is telling them that it is such a crime, they say, 'No one's, it's just my own. It's just how I am.' This is because it has become so deeply ingrained, they don't stop to think about whether it is true or not. Their unconscious still sees these rules as a matter of life or death, even though as adults their survival is predicated on much more complicated matters than pleasing their parents, and even when the voice continuing the mantra is their own.

Some family 'rules' even manifest physically: perhaps you are the tall one in your family, which makes someone else in the family feel inadequate, so in order to fit in better and not aggravate them, you learn to hunch your shoulders slightly so as not to stand out. Your body becomes very used to this posture and you don't even know you are doing it. Telling you to stand up straight won't make any difference because to you that hunched feeling *is* what standing up straight feels like.

Or perhaps you were told off if you complained of being tired, or you heard others being derided for being lazy. You may have absorbed from this the notion that you have to ignore your tiredness and just power on through no matter what. Your mind stops recognising the signals that your body is sending you as it tries to tell you that you are too tired. You push and you push until your body gets completely overloaded and forces you to stop through illness or injury, or your neglected spouse leaves you.

Such early-learned patterns are difficult to overcome, and for those of you who weren't given permission to ever really notice and make allowances for your own needs, letting self-compassion in now can take time. You may need to defy years of conditioning to let yourself do so. Or even to see the need to do so. A therapist can help you work on this reluctance, gently unravelling the messages that you've absorbed, bringing them into consciousness where they can be re-examined in the light of new, adult information. But sometimes even then you will only grasp the idea intellectually; absorbing this new information into your body takes longer. This is how yoga can help you take them on board in a non-verbal, non-intellectual, non-brain-driven way. The way

Find Some Compassion

Dominique puts it is that the balance she eventually found was 'unexplainable'.

Letting Compassion In

Your yoga practice provides the time and space to start listening in to your body on a micro level. This sends the message that you are doing things differently now. Dominique says she was able to unlearn old patterns. She did it, and you can do it, by showing your body that you care, which is half the battle. The other half is allowing it to be how it is, rather than judging it and telling it you would prefer it to be different. Something that may help you get on board with this notion is understanding one of the main philosophies that underpins the yogic approach to life. This is a concept called *ahimsa*, which means non-violence or non-harming. As with all things yogic, this notion works on many levels – practical and conceptual, physical and emotional; and it applies not just to others but also to yourself.

On a practical level, obviously we want to be careful not to harm our bodies by pushing ourselves to the point of injury. And we could just as easily harm ourselves emotionally, if we are constantly bullying our body to do things it isn't ready for, or with constant criticism that we should be doing better or going further, or comparison to others, or to our younger selves.

By undertaking a commitment to practise *ahimsa*, to not be violent, you need to include yourself. If you are pushing yourself beyond what your body is prepared to tolerate, if you are constantly criticising yourself, if you are alienating friends, then you are not practising *ahimsa*. If you are not practising *ahimsa* then you are not really doing yoga, you are merely exercising, and you are repeating old, familiar habits and patterns that are not going to transform you in any meaningful way. Instead, practising *ahimsa* means you are gently encouraging and trying out a different approach.

Similarly, in psychotherapy your therapist will gently question how much your old habits are helping you and how much they are hindering you. One approach in particular – the person-centred approach to psychotherapy, founded by Carl Rogers – seems to me to have a lot of parallels to the notion of *ahimsa*.

Rogers felt that for a person to grow and become all they could be – to 'self-actualise'[7] – they need an environment in which three core conditions are met: empathy, congruence and unconditional positive regard. Empathy I think most of us will understand as listening and being listened to and understood kindly; congruence is the harmony between what you feel to be true and what is said to be true; while unconditional positive regard means accepting and being accepted as you are, flaws and all.

Both empathy and unconditional positive regard are akin to the notion of *ahimsa*, and to the sort of qualities we are trying to evoke and engender in our yoga practice. For instance, you can apply unconditional positive regard by not beating yourself up because you need a prop to get into a yoga pose when no one else in class does and you can tell yourself you are doing a really positive thing just by being there, no matter what poses you do or don't do while there.

Allowing some self-compassion into your practice, then, not only means you are honouring the traditional spirit of yoga, but also that you are giving yourself the same conditions for growth that a psychotherapist would offer as part of your psychotherapy. Given that both Eastern and Western traditions value self-compassion so highly, are you able to reframe the idea of self-pity as self-compassion and try it out occasionally?

Find Some Compassion

Human nature being what it is, I can almost hear the pushback – a positive cacophony of 'yes, buts…'.

Barriers to Self-Compassion

'Yes, but' is a classic response that emerges almost instantly when we are faced with a notion that challenges our internal working model. We immediately leap to focusing on all the reasons why doing things differently won't work. Please may I try to pre-empt some of your 'yes-buts' with a bit more explanation?

We have to become consciously aware of our internal working models if we are to have a chance of changing them. But even after our therapist and/or our yoga practice have helped us with this, we then have to deal with the defences that will try to stop our attempts at dismantling them. They are so deeply ingrained, so much a part of who we think we are, that all that we hold dear – our very personalities – can seem as if it's under attack. By which I mean that as soon as they are challenged, one of our critical internal voices will immediately find the loophole that explains why changing would be a terrible idea.

I'm guessing that around about now one of your critical voices might be saying, *'That's all very well, but I can't let myself off the hook that easily; if I loosen the reins at all, that lazy, victim-ey* [add whatever your own personal critical script is here] *part of me will just run riot, I'll never get it back under control and everyone will hate me and talk about me behind my back.'* Or it might be saying a cleverer and more grown-up version of the above; but basically a variation on it. There are many possible responses to this, but here are two for now:

First, contemporary academic researchers such as Kristin Neff and Dr Chris Germer of Harvard Medical School have been discovering a scientific basis to the value of self-compassion[8], as well as indications that increasing self-compassion leads to greater compassion for others. Neff and Germer's research shows that when it comes to making big life changes, self-compassion is actually the greatest source of strength you have to draw on because it provides the supportive emotional environment without which change is impossible. It also shows that those who are hard on themselves are less resilient after a setback and more prone to mental-health issues. So:

- self-compassion works – the ancient yogis have been saying this for years based on their experience and now scientists can see it via measurable modern means.
- if you can be nicer to yourself, you will be nicer to others.

So if for no other reason, do it for those around you – it would be selfish not to! And bear in mind that a judgement about someone else is generally really a judgement about yourself. Learn not to judge yourself and you learn not to judge others so harshly.

My second response is to acknowledge that, yes, if you go completely to the opposite end of the spectrum and allow yourself 'everything', then there is a risk that you may get stuck there, indulging in endless metaphorical duvet days. And that is no better than being stuck at the self-critical end. More later about this tendency to think that we cannot allow ourselves an inch or we will take a mile, but for now, I will simply say that all of this is why we need self-awareness to guide us towards a realistic balance.

Much of therapy is about finding balance, and yoga is pretty much defined by it, finding equilibrium between those two extremes of not allowing yourself anything versus allowing yourself everything (which isn't actually compassionate anyway). It is possible to find a middle path.

My suggestions to help encourage some self-compassion are:

Find Some Compassion

- **Practise *metta* meditation**

There is more to come about meditation, but one meditation practice that focuses specifically on igniting compassion is called *metta*, or loving-kindness meditation. This flexes your compassion muscle towards others and, in turn, towards yourself. Research has measured and proved the effectiveness of this type of meditation on increasing levels of compassion and many yogis have noticed this happening through their own experience, often discovering that it brings up quite a lot of emotion along with it.[9]

- **Set self-compassion as your intention**

It is common in yoga to set an intention at the start of a class or session. This focuses the mind on why you are practising, encouraging you to stay present and reminding you that you are connecting to something broader than the purely physical. An intention can be whatever you want it to be and can be aimed at yourself, at someone else or at the world in general. It can be specific or general. Try setting greater self-compassion as your intention from time to time and see what happens when you dedicate your practice to yourself in this way.

- **Discover yoga philosophy**

Learn about *ahimsa* and the other yogic precepts and – if they resonate with you – see if you can embody them as part of your practice. Not only can their lessons be life-enhancing, but practising in this way connects you to yoga's more philosophical aspects, which could deepen your practice. If it doesn't appeal, then don't worry; however you engage with it, yoga will speak to you and help you in many ways. However, if you are so inclined, connecting to the teachings through the historical texts and their modern interpretations could make your yoga more meaningful and thus give you more reasons to do it, be more fulfilling when you do so and provide closer integration of mind, body and spirit. Many good teachers and studios incorporate some of these teachings in their classes.

- **Practise yin yoga**

Much of the yoga done in the West has what Chinese philosophy would categorise as a yang energy – vigorous, fast-paced, aimed at igniting or keeping us in a state dominated by the sympathetic nervous system, often focused on 'achievement'. But as we are finding out, this needs to be balanced with what the Chinese would call yin energy, aimed at cooling and slowing. So you need a practice that speaks to that equally great need to activate our parasympathetic nervous system, where calmness and kindness can reside.

Yin yoga is one of several modern approaches to yoga that recognise the prevailing Western, twenty-first-century tendency to deprioritise this, and offer something different.

Unlike more active approaches, which work mainly on strengthening and stretching the muscles, yin yoga aims to work on the deep connective tissues – the fascia, tendons and ligaments that, in anatomical terms, are more about stabilising, holding and nourishing. Think about the symbolism of those functions – can you apply it more generally to your life's priorities and needs?

The yin approach is gentle and compassion-focused and aims to ignite sensation and deepen awareness while allowing deep rest and relaxation, softening the body and providing a break from all the pushing and achieving. Yin focuses on the more floor-based postures, asking that you stay in them for longer periods of time. Physically this gives rarely used tissues the chance to stretch and lengthen; mentally it gives you a chance to really notice and observe how you feel, actively choose a more compassionate response and attitude to yourself.

Find Some Compassion

I have two final thoughts about self-compassion to leave you with. When we feel or offer compassion to others we don't tend to see it as offering them pity; rather, we feel genuinely moved by their suffering and understand them to be deserving of warmth and care. And yet if we think of behaving like this towards ourselves, we so often re-label it as self-pity. I often ask my therapy clients to conjure up a picture of themselves when they were smaller and younger. Can you do this and then imagine subjecting this you, or a beloved friend, to the kind of thoughts and behaviour that you apply to yourself as an adult? Can you see how cruel and brutal this now feels?

My second thought is that we tend to think of compassion as a zero-sum game, whereby we only have a limited amount to go round, and that if any goes towards ourselves we will have less to offer others. However, all the research says that the opposite is true – the more we have, the more we can generate – so offering it to yourself will strengthen your ability to offer it to others. As Dominique says – now she can love herself, and her community. One will encourage the other.

Yoga Saved My Life
Elizabeth Luna

Diagnosed with breast cancer two months after my stepson's suicide, my spirit was crushed.

I remained strong for the sake of my family, internalising my own grief with the help of prescription drugs to numb the pain. Grieving made me question everything, including my spiritual faith.

After my bilateral mastectomy and reconstruction surgeries I suffered from intense anxiety and depression. I was angry and I felt cheated and robbed of my femininity.

I constantly struggled with whether my husband would find me attractive without breasts and whether I would love myself without them. My perception of myself changed and I continually battled with negative inner chatter.

With two years of therapy I began mentally adjusting to my new body and learning how to live again.

But it wasn't until practising yoga consistently that I truly began my physical, spiritual and healing journey.

Yoga makes me feel complete and not separated from myself. It allows me to heal emotional trauma. The movements heal my wounds each time I practise and it changes my negative thoughts into positive thinking.

It improved my health during recovery when I could barely raise my arms to my head and, most importantly, it improved my desire to heal depression and anxiety. Yoga gives me more confidence to share my feelings and not internalise them.

Intentions and Philosophies

Earlier I talked of the yogic custom of setting an intention at the start of each practice. My own intention for this book is to aim for inclusivity and accessibility, and that means I often find myself minimising references to the more esoteric and complex elements of yogic philosophy.

Find Some Compassion

However, it is important to know that those deeper levels exist because they are integral to why yoga is not just exercise plus relaxation, and why it can be so life-changing.

Yoga consists of different teachings from different eras and from different lineages – yoga belongs to no one era, place or person. Much is common and universal, but each lineage and approach has its own particular take on how best to conceptualise the world we live in, our place in it, and how we function as human beings.

The notion of *ahimsa* originates, it is thought, from the *Yoga Sutras*, written by, it is thought, a sage called Patanjali.

The *Sutras* offer guidelines, a road map, as to how to live a life that is healthy, satisfying, ethical, and which will connect you to something greater than yourself. For instance, its ten best known 'disciplines and habits' consist of the following:

Ahimsa – not harming in word, thought or deed
Satya – not lying, i.e. honesty
Asteya – not stealing
Brahmacharya – using creative energy for higher purposes
Aparigraha – not being greedy or hoarding
Saucha – cleanliness and purity
Santosha – contentment
Tapas – discipline and minimalist existence
Svadhyaya – introspection, self-study, textual study
Isvara Pranidhana – contemplation of a higher power.

In these ten codes you can probably also see the parallels to Christianity's Ten Commandments (but without the 'commanding' element), to Buddhism's Ten Virtues and, more generally, to the things that most of us contemplate, aim for or struggle with in our everyday lives. They are the themes that lie behind much of what I see clients bringing into my therapy room and they underpin many of the Fierce Calm stories we've been hearing.

Deepening your enquiry and engaging with the philosophies takes yoga off the mat and weaves it into the very fabric of your life.

Another of my intentions in this book is to draw parallels between what I, a Western psychotherapist, find yoga can do for me and my clients, and comparing this with what I find psychotherapy can do for us. It is about exploring how closely the two mirror each other. But that does not mean this is the only way to understand the human condition. Yogic philosophy offers alternative conceptualisations as to how and why we do what we do and is well worth investigating further.

Explore any route that interests you, draw your inspiration from anything that resonates and makes sense to you and keep an open mind towards understanding that we are all 'works in progress', each of us finding our own ways of being in the world with whatever resources are available to us and via whichever approach makes most sense to us. Yoga's different lineages, psychotherapy's different approaches, all have something to offer. Explore and find what works for you.

If you want others to be happy, practise compassion. If you want to be happy, practise compassion.

The Dalai Lama

CHAPTER FIVE

You Can't Pour From an Empty Cup

Yoga Saved My Life
Enricka Shanté

As an only child I struggled with feeling alone. When I was fourteen my mother, who had had multiple miscarriages, told me she was pregnant. I was excited but also fearful of more loss. When I was sixteen I was left to take care of my brother while my mom worked multiple jobs to make ends meet.

I started having unhealthy and unloving thoughts, sometimes cutting myself. I witnessed physical and verbal abuse I didn't know how to process. At twenty-two my little brother died in a tragic accident and I lost all hope.

I wanted to die, wishing I could take my mother's pain away, wishing I could stop my own pain. I lost my first love due to my depression and unwillingness to see a brighter future.

I turned back to my faith, but something was still missing. So, I went searching. I discovered yoga.

I kept trying to find love and validation through others. When I found yoga it started to clear my thoughts and

> made me want to expand and be open to all the possibilities. It allowed me to love myself. I was able to shift my perspective. I learned to let go of what wasn't serving me. I still have to work through my depression every day, but yoga helps me through all the sticky stuff that holds me back. Let go of what you must so that you can grow to love yourself.

This chapter follows on very neatly from the one on compassion and is closely allied to it. We are going to ponder the notion of self-care. This too springs from one of the most common things that I hear in my therapy room: the sense of guilt that coming to therapy evokes because it is seen as a self-indulgence. To take one whole hour out of the one hundred and sixty-eight hours in a week to pause and spend some time exploring your feelings! Such decadence! The same is often said of incorporating a yoga practice into a busy life. We tend sometimes to label both therapy and yoga as selfish and unjustified; as with the idea of self-compassion, we see ourselves as undeserving of this time spent on ourselves.

This idea upsets me as it is not only cruel and self-abusive, but actually counterproductive. We can only help others if we first help ourselves. There is a reason that airline staff tell us to put our own oxygen masks on first. If we are depleted, weak and not 'there' for ourselves, how can we possibly be there for others? This is obviously not the only reason to think about yourself, but it is often the only way I can make it palatable to people allergic to self-care notions.

There is a concept called 'emotional contagion',[10] which has shown that feelings are catching. This makes it all the more important that what we transmit to others is replenishing rather than draining. This will also give us more tools to avoid being 'infected' by the poor emotional state of others who may be the very reason we feel the need to prioritise them at the expense of ourselves. See how easy it can be for a vicious circle to get set up and then become entrenched? But equally, a virtuous circle could so easily take its place if we *allow* ourselves to self-care.

Survival of the Nurtured

The word 'allowing' is a useful one; we need to look at why and how it might be so difficult for us to allow ourselves self-nurture. What feels 'allowed' in terms of taking time for us? In terms of saying 'I deserve this'? Why is that so hard? Louis Cozolino, a psychiatrist and professor of interpersonal neurobiology, studies the intersection of mind, body, brain and relationships. He has discovered that good relationships and a healthy sense of self can actually cause new neural pathways in the brain to grow.[11] As a result of this he has come up with the memorable claim – defying Darwin – that we thrive not due to survival of the fittest but by survival of the nurtured.

So, far from being an optional, indulgent luxury, self-nurture is, in fact, life-saving and a way to relate to oneself in a more positive and constructive way that will reduce trauma and increase connection to others.

Yet we resist. A psychotherapist will help you look back at the conditions in which this viewpoint was able to take root and work with you to understand which experiences led to this lack of self-worth that makes you feel not deserving of care. In therapy you can pick away at the 'truths' behind this belief and work to repair the faulty notion of self. We have previously looked at whose voice might be telling you that you are not worthy; with your therapist you may be able to better identify the source of this critical voice, see it for what it is and start to find a substitute voice that can offer a counterview.

Therapy is often described as a reparative environment, which means that the relationship between therapist and client can offer an alternative experience of care, allowing you to discover a different version of yourself, a more valuable, a more loved version, and thus transform.

We can see from Enricka's experience that yoga can do a similar job. She tells us how learning to love herself through yoga was the starting point that allowed her to expand and find possibilities. How can yoga do this?

One way is through the yoga community in general and your teacher or teachers in particular. There can be something reparative about the yoga community that is similar to that of a good relationship. It can offer a different experience of a world that is not all about criticism, but that sees self-enquiry, self-compassion and self-acceptance as necessary for survival. In yoga we often find a less punishing 'tribe' into which we can be welcomed. Yoga, and particularly the notion of *ahimsa* (non-violence or non-harming), can formalise and give permission for a way of accepting yourself that may be the polar opposite to the way you tried to make yourself acceptable as a child. It can feed back a different voice, a less critical, more nurturing voice, which tells you not only that you are allowed to spend this time on yourself, but that you are acceptable just as you are. It can give you the courage to say no to things you don't want to do and yes to those you do.

Again, this does not mean just giving yourself permission to lie around doing nothing all the time. Even a challenging yoga practice can be done compassionately, without harshness, and done instead with acceptance as to what is possible for you today, as opposed to focusing on achievement. Achievement in yoga comes when you can listen, accept and allow, not when you can get your ankle behind your head.

Another way in which yoga provides a reparative environment is that it can increase your ability to quieten the critical voice inside and turn up the volume on the nurturing voice, allowing you to befriend your body, deem it worthy of care, come to see it as an equal partner in your decision-making. You can learn to stop pushing it about as though it were a piece of furniture. The truth is that your body will give you so much more if it feels loved. As the Dalai Lama teaches, affection is an antidote to fear.[12] When a person is kind to us, we feel we can trust them, so we relax. The same is true for our muscles, which will soften and give more if they feel safe.

There is also another more pragmatic reason to make friends with your body, which is that it has valuable information to offer, as we will come to learn.

There are many ways in which you can use your yoga practice to look after yourself and put fuel back in the tank. For a start, just giving yourself space in your day to do something for yourself is a really important acknowledgement that you matter, that you value yourself enough to take care of your body and mind. A regular, *ahimsa*-informed yoga practice can provide a formal structure that might feel more permissible. It's almost like a behavioural-therapy approach – do the behaviour often enough and it starts to feel acceptable; the self-care muscle strengthens. If your tank is constantly being emptied without being refilled, it will very soon be drained and therefore useless and unable to provide anything for you – or anyone else.

So take some time each day to stop, check in and give yourself what you need.

- **Make the time**
Reframe your yoga practice as a refuelling stop, a necessary few minutes in the day to drink in its oxygen and allow yourself to be replenished, knowing you will go back out stronger and with more to give. The kind of replenishment you need will vary from day to day, so the first task is to listen compassionately to what your body requires in the moment

- **Choose wisely**
Once on your mat, you have the choice to either challenge or go easy on yourself, depending on what you need that day. So check in. Notice how you feel, pay attention to what your body is telling you (not your mind) and only then decide – honestly – what is most nurturing for today. Having decided on your approach your next choice is what type of practice best fits with those needs. Ideally, a practice will give you a bit of everything and take you seamlessly to and fro across a line between energising and calming, challenging your notion of what is possible and softening you into poses to recharge and nurture you. But remember that you can also gear your session more towards activity or passivity, depending on the day's need. Whatever you end up choosing to do, do it compassionately and with self-care. Part of that self-care is to make sure you start by checking in with, and warming up, each body part in turn.

- **Limber and listen**
Most of us understand the need to warm up the body physiologically before putting it through demanding exercise. But rather than seeing this as a boring necessity to be half-heartedly 'got through' before the real exercise begins, try to bring a caring and enquiring mind to each individual part of the

body. Start to see your body as an integral part of you that has great wisdom to offer, not as a separate 'thing' that you 'do things' to. Yoga in general, and the limbering up in particular, asks us to give each body part its due care and attention. I see parallels here with a therapist trying to understand the everyday, habitual patterns and behaviours that may seem insignificant and yet might give clues as to where the bigger issues originated.

Try to get as microscopic as you can with your limbering up; alongside moving the larger muscles like hamstrings, quads, biceps, triceps and so on, focus minutely on the parts of your body that many of us tend not to notice or appreciate so much – the ankles, wrists, individual toes and fingers. It's so easy to overlook and take these for granted, yet these are often the parts we use and rely on most. Break a finger or sprain an ankle and you very quickly realise just how crucial the smaller parts are to the overall whole.

Here are some thoughts as to what really focusing on the warm-up might look like in practice:

- Try scrunching up all your toes and then spreading them wide. Can you separate them or do some seem fused together? Can you move each individually?
- What happens when you curl up your foot and then stretch it out? Can you now feel the arch? Are you ever normally aware of the arch?
- Can you draw a circle with your ankle? Can you feel if some parts get stuck, or are painful, or maybe can't be felt at all?
- And what about each individual vertebra in your spine? Each one has an important job to play, as well as contributing to the whole. The cat/cow sequence (*bitilasana marjaryasana*) is popular as a warm-up in yoga classes and books. This movement

of the back takes the full length of the spine – crown to tailbone – from a back-bending movement to a forward-bending one. Slow this down. Try to feel which vertebrae move easily and which seem stuck.

Explore, listen and bring empathy to each body part. If possible, bring gratitude too; appreciate what every element, however tiny, brings to the party and acknowledge its contribution. Show all parts of yourself the same thoughtfulness.

Caring for your body, for yourself, is an important way to spot mistakes before they happen. Think about how engineers, sailors, racing-car drivers, fishermen, anyone who works with machines or vehicles, all have to keep every rope, every cog, every wheel oiled and cared for. Your body is your vehicle and needs the same consideration.

Paying attention to even small body parts with compassion and care shows your body, shows your very soul, that every little bit of you matters; that the whole team cannot function happily if just one member of the crew is sick or neglected. The small things can very easily become larger things – the arch of a foot that repeatedly collapses rather than lifts can lead to the growth of a bunion, which then pushes the whole foot off balance, causing the leg to place pressure in the wrong areas, which pushes the hip and sacrum out of balance to counteract the droop… and hey presto, you have a bad back that goes on for years and defies all attempts to 'cure' it because the back is not where the problem originated. So too with our depression, our anxiety, our moodiness, our anger, our general unhappiness – these things began with us ignoring the little niggle, the 'too-silly-to-mention' slight that stung, the tiredness we didn't acknowledge, the injustice we felt or the fear that we were embarrassed by. Pay attention to the small things with love and the big things won't have a chance to grow – in the body as in the mind.

- **Explore restorative yoga**

Restorative yoga is deeply relaxing. It uses props like bolsters and cushions and nurturing items like an eye pillow to keep out the light and blankets to keep you warm. It largely involves lying still, supported by these props, so that you can allow your body to completely release and are thus able to let go of any tension, any need to move. It promotes deep rest, sometimes even sleep.

As you can see, the suggestions in this chapter are really all about preparation and attitude. Checking in with your bodymind – your physical self, your emotional self, your caring self, as well as your thinking self – and listening, paying attention and responding kindly to it, will enhance any type of practice; and those lessons learned on the mat will soon start to be absorbed into your life off the mat, just as the lessons learned in therapy soon start to be internalised and accessible outside the therapy room.

Refuelling Your Own Tank

If, for example, you are a carer for someone else, if you are a parent, or have elderly parents, or work in the caring professions, you will be doubly susceptible to the notion that you do not deserve self-compassion and self-care, because you can always see others who have it worse, or who are more in need. But imagine you had a broken arm – meeting someone with two broken arms might make you feel sympathy for them and gratitude that you at least have one working arm, but it doesn't make your own broken one hurt any less.

There will always be people worse off than you, but that doesn't make your own pain unworthy of attention. You are allowed to tend your own wounds, refuel your own tank. You will be better able to help others, as well as yourself, if you do. Amanda tells us in her story later on that yoga enabled her to breathe life into a soul that felt crushed from years of caretaking, enabling her to better help those who needed her by finding love and joy in herself.

Lack of self-compassion and self-care is often behind many of the other issues we will be looking at throughout this book. So making time to incorporate a compassionate yoga practice into your life is a great place to embark on your journey to better self-knowledge and all the health and emotional benefits it brings.

Top-down and Bottom-up

We've seen that the bodymind is one unified entity, but we've also seen how sometimes, when the communication channels are not working brilliantly, the brain and body can occasionally work against, rather than for, each other, and that one can come to unhelpfully dominate the other – like your head telling your body to override its needs for recuperation, or your body manifesting illness so as to get rest it would otherwise not be allowed.

One way of conceptualising the complex messaging system throughout the bodymind is to think in terms of the predominant direction of travel of these messages.

Top-Down Processing
Top-down or efferent processing is when the brain sends messages downwards to the body. This includes useful

and valuable things like the brain telling the body to lift a cup, to scratch an itch, to get itself out of a difficult situation. Top-down processing is also what throws you a flotation device when you feel overwhelmed by emotions that threaten to drown you. It can be a life raft that enables you to engage your brain and tell yourself that you can survive whatever has just happened, lets you understand that your random behaviour is a normal response to something, that you do have resources and agency and skills that can help.

Less useful are the top-down messages that tell the body to ignore its tiredness and have a cup of coffee instead of taking a rest. Unfortunately, modern society and working practices generally favour this form of processing, reward us for it even. We think we can override pain or hunger or fear through sheer force of will. We then turn up in our therapist's office unable to feel anything from the neck down, wanting solutions but not understanding that it is by connecting to our feelings that the real work of transformation can begin.

Bottom-Up Processing
Bottom-up, or afferent, processing is when the body sends messages upwards to the brain.

Useful and valuable bottom-up responses include your stomach telling you it needs food, or your legs telling you it's time to sit down and stop walking; and those which happen before you've realised it – your hand jumping back from a flame.

Bottom-up messages are not so useful when unregulated feelings of anger result in you punching someone, or sadness paralyses you into not getting out of bed for three days, or causing you to eat a whole tub of ice cream.

We do need both systems, though, and when afferent and efferent are in balance then it's a cooperative partnership, each 'end' of the bodymind keeping the other informed and suggesting actions that keep the whole system functioning optimally.

But as we have seen, it doesn't work quite so harmoniously when one half of the partnership gets carried away. And, more often than not, it is the brain that tends to take charge. It forgets that the body has valuable information to offer, and it stops listening, overriding messages of hunger or tiredness, fear or sadness. This is why learning to listen to your body and treating it as an equal partner in the decision-making process is so essential.

Yoga and our processing systems
Yoga provides the perfect feedback loop to enable us to develop the skills to improve communication between top-down and bottom-up messages.

It helps top-down processing through the practices of meditation, chanting and teaching us how to better observe what it is we are doing, so strengthening awareness rather than just acting on automatic pilot – developing what's known as the observer self (more on that later). As our thoughts become clearer and we are better able to reappraise and reframe an unnecessarily stressed or panicked state, we are sending a crucial message of clear-headedness downwards, which will reassure and soothe an anxious body into believing a 'grown up' is in charge who won't panic.

Yoga equally strengthens bottom-up processing, by encouraging embodiment – a better connection with the body – while also deepening the sense of grounding and being more anchored to the Earth. This gets us in touch with, and more familiar with, the body – what it is saying and what it needs. Learning to listen to, interpret and act on these messages from the body can influence the mind, tempering its propensity to arrogance and dictatorialism and allowing more collaboration between afferent and efferent systems.

Yoga teaches us to discern when it is more useful to allow the skills of the brain to take the lead, and when those of the body are in a better place to do so instead. It has been proven to have measurable effects on the bodily warning signals such as heart and respiration rates,[13] thus reducing our chances of heart attack, stroke and more.

Psychotherapy and our processing systems
In therapy too we learn how to allow ourselves to both think and feel our way into our issues. We start to use our cognition alongside our feelings, and thereby incorporate and integrate all aspects of our personalities.

Psychotherapy works both in a top-down way by 'educating' the brain into clearer ways of thinking and message-sending, and it works bottom-up by providing the experience of a nurturing relationship. Within a trusting relationship the feelings that might seem terrifying or overwhelming when alone can emerge safely.

Yoga Saved My Life
Amanda Stetler

My husband was diagnosed with incurable cancer and overnight I was thrust into a life of unknowns.

Riddled with anxiety, I would find myself unable to breathe yet trying to bury the internal panic to better support my husband and our three children under four years old.

Yoga had always been something I had practised, but it now became my anchor. Finding strength and mindfulness on my mat gave me strength and mindfulness in the crazy life that was my existence.

My husband has had no reprieve from his cancer battle. But yoga gives life and purpose to the valuable hours and minutes and seconds of each day. It breathed life into a soul that felt crushed, making me human again, able to love and feel joy despite the darkness.

We made big life changes, including a move across the country to a home that provided the healing elements and the calm of nature.

My daily practice has become a guiding light to my walk as a caregiver, wife, mother and teacher, helping me to show gratitude with each present moment of life. Together, this family is living life fiercely, loving deeply and finding peace together.

Body and soul are not two substances but one. They are man becoming aware of himself in two different ways.

C. F. Von Weizsacher

CHAPTER SIX

Finding Strength

Yoga Saved My Life
Brienna Drees

Two years ago my brother's lifeless body was found hanging in the basement of our house. I watched my entire family fall apart. I spent every day bawling my eyes out, stuffing the covers in my mouth because my cries were so loud. I barely graduated high school, I even turned to drugs and alcohol. I fell into a deep depression and fought for my life every single day. I broke down at the sight of ambulances that led to horrible flashbacks and nightmares of losing my best friend.

I spent my Friday nights in the cemetery because sitting at my brother's grave sounded better than being with friends. I was so lost; some days I still am.

Saying yoga saved me is an understatement. My mat was the only place I could peacefully cry and release the horrible images that rest inside my head every day. Breath and meditation allowed me to visualise my brother floating among the cosmos, happy and finally home.

The comfort and strength I've found within myself, because of yoga, has allowed me to conquer every day and

> become a light for myself and others. It has allowed me to be reborn and find peace in the chaos.
>
> Yoga saved my life and my entire soul.

Do you ever feel like there's just too much to cope with? Many of my clients are brought to therapy by that sense of overwhelm and confusion about all that they are 'meant' to be doing, their inability to keep on top of it all and the feeling they are doing many things badly as opposed to one thing well.

Physically, they are easy to spot. All their energy is fluttering around their upper chest and throat, they breathe shallowly, they seem untethered and flighty, flitting from idea to idea, task to task in a superficial way, unable to settle and deal with anything properly. Like a circus performer trying to spin too many plates, they stay on their toes so they can run from one to the other, never settling and with all the plates forever on the brink, mere seconds away from collapse. And sometimes they do collapse – not being able to cope can also manifest as complete shutdown and defeat.

But while still spinning, this person can never come to stillness, can never put a full foot on the ground; they have to always remain primed and ready to run to the next about-to-topple plate. To put it simply, they are unconnected to the ground and, just like those flying plates, share only a glancing connection with the stability it could provide.

Yoga can help us find some necessary solidity, in a very practical and concrete way. A class or session starts with finding the floor – literally – whether by lying down on the floor, feeling our feet on the ground or sitting or kneeling down. Finding our anchor is very important in psychotherapeutic terms too.

Finding Strength

A Secure Base

As we saw earlier, John Bowlby's psychotherapeutic approach termed attachment theory[14] recognises that we all have an innate need for an emotionally secure base. Without a secure base, a solid starting point, we can feel unconnected, adrift, fragmented and overwhelmed. Without a secure base we cannot explore and grow.

In therapy you might look at why you feel so unanchored, and work towards seeking out people and new ways of being that can help you connect and feel more secure in your base.

In yoga, we can literally and physically connect with a base – the Earth – in different ways depending on our energy levels and our needs that day.

- **Grounding**

Some days lying down might feel like the best way to anchor yourself. It gives you the largest possible surface area available to be in contact with the ground. Physically feeling this solid base beneath the full length of your body allows you to release down into it, absorbing the sensation of being supported, of not having to hold yourself up.

Other days you may feel panicked by all that you are 'failing' in. If so, starting your practice by lying on your back doing very little may just reinforce your feelings of failure. Or it may cause stress at the idea that you are floating into a relaxation that will not help you energise and engage with all that you need to get on and 'do'. On those days a standing practice may better help ground and fortify you.

When standing, only the soles of your feet are in contact with the floor – not a very large area considering how much of you it is holding upright. So you really need to feel confident about your feet being well connected. In the balancing postures section earlier I suggested closing your eyes and focusing your attention on the soles, imagining the feet growing wider and more stable. A similar visualisation could be useful here:

- As the soles of the feet expand in your imagination, envisage them sprouting little tentacles, roots, that are reaching down into the solid earth below. Just as the roots of a tree reach not only downwards but also out wide in a huge diameter, so too your roots are reaching wide as well as deep.
- Visualise these roots spreading out wider and burrowing ever deeper until you sense a broad, solid base that holds you tight and connects you to the depths of the Earth. The Earth that will never let you down, will always be there as an anchor to return to.
- Let your weight drop down into that support. Give in to gravity as you feel the pull of your roots drawing your spine and its weight down into the earth.
- If it's still hard to feel anchored, then try putting a little bend in your knees as this can help drop the weight downwards.

This may all feel a bit like collapse, this notion of being pulled down. You may wonder – 'Isn't this feeling of everything dragging me down the very thing I'm trying to combat?' Well, yes, but remember that yoga is always about uniting opposites, or what appear to be opposites. In order to go up we need to go down first. Think of a trampoline: if you just stand on it and try to jump up, you will not reach very high. But if you press down first, use the gravitational downward force to get some momentum, then you will jump higher. A bird pushes its wing down to gain momentum

Finding Strength

to take it up. This principle is true of all yoga poses – you can't go skywards without first reaching 'ground-wards'. It is the deep connection with your support that will propel you higher.

So having forged that relationship with the ground, felt its solidity, tested that your roots are strong, now you have a secure base from which to reach up and achieve your potential: the sky's the limit. Feet firmly rooted, allow the crown of your head to reach for infinity where nothing can hold you back. Feel your upper body drawn upwards, creating space and lightness emotionally, and also practically, in that your spine lengthening upwards in this way creates space for each vertebra.

I like imagery and metaphor, and there is an image that helps me with this idea of grounding. It couldn't be more un-yogic, but it nevertheless helps me feel more solid. Those of you who grew up in the seventies might remember a children's toy called a Weeble that looked like a painted egg. There was an annoyingly catchy advertising jingle that went 'Weebles wobble but they don't fall down'. This is because a Weeble was heavily weighted in the base, which meant that no matter which way you pushed it, it would always spring back up. It was really in touch with where its centre of gravity was.

I don't know if summoning up your inner Weeble will help you in the way it does me, but if there is a similar image that works for you, use it to help you bring a sense of rootedness to your practice and know – and feel – that the more secure your base, the better you will cope.

- **Standing postures**

All yoga postures rely on a solid connection with the Earth, but the standing postures really drive the point home, dependent as they are on a solid grounding through your feet. The most fundamental of all – *tadasana* (mountain pose) – says it all with its name. You can become like a mountain, immovable and connected to a broad base. It may look like a simple posture, just something to transition through to the more 'exciting' ones. But learning to stand, learning to ground yourself, to find that anchor, can be not only one of the hardest poses to inhabit, but also one of the most necessary. When my husband, Bill, died, I didn't know which way was up. Everything I thought I could rely on, even the very ground upon which I stood, felt like it had betrayed me, and like a small child I had to learn to stand and walk again. One of my beloved yoga teachers, Catherine Annis, helped me to do this in the weeks after Bill's unexpected death. She helped me regain my *tadasana*, my inner mountain, my connection to the Earth. That was pretty much all we did for several sessions – she helped me learn to stand upright again, find a secure base.

Another symbolic and grounding standing pose is *asvatasana* – horse pose. The wide-leg stance reinforces the sense of solidity and stability. The bended knees take your centre of gravity lower (think of sumo wrestlers). A dynamic version of *asvatasana* will move you effortlessly between the two polarities. Reaching downwards, you anchor your base in the earth, staying connected there while extending your arms up into the air as a reminder that you can also reach skywards, the world your oyster, nourished from above and below: solid and dependable below the waist, light and free above.

On a more physical level, this posture builds enormous strength in the thighs, alongside a more symbolic buttressing – I am solid, I can hold this pose, I can cope. Brienna words echo this when she tells us of the comfort and strength she found within herself, the peace in the chaos.

Utkatasana, chair pose, has similarly good grounding qualities. Again, the bent knees lower the centre of gravity, reinforcing the connection to the ground in the lower body, strengthening the legs, feet and ankles, all while the upper body floats skywards towards its potential.

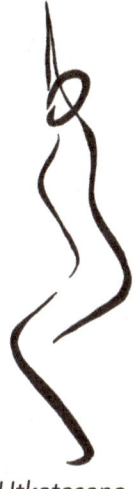

Utkatasana

The Vagus Nerve

The vagus nerve is pretty much the largest motorway in the body's network. It connects the brain to a myriad other organs ('vagus' comes from the same root word as 'vagabond', meaning wanderer, which gives you an indication of how far-reaching its route throughout the body is). A huge 80 per cent of the information this nerve carries is afferent – bottom-up – sending messages to the brain about the body's need for food, safety, rest and so much more.

A well-functioning vagus nerve is said to be 'toned'. This can be measured via what is known as heart-rate variability or HRV (the time interval between consecutive heartbeats). Many studies[15] have shown just how crucial yoga is for improving vagal tone and heart-rate variability, which has implications for heart health and respiratory rate. But its effects go way beyond the physical. Ground-breaking research by scientist and professor of psychiatry Stephen Porges has led to a new and compelling theory, which is proving massively influential to both yoga and psychotherapy. It is known as polyvagal theory because it recognises that there are two sides to the vagus nerve – dorsal and ventral – and that these influence our nervous system in very different ways, both of which affect how we respond to stress and trauma.

The ventral vagus has recently been found[16] to be a very important factor in our ability to socialise and connect with others. This has huge implications psychologically. The more toned this branch of the nerve, the more able we are to allow others to help soothe us, which has massive repercussions for our ability to respond to things like stress, anxiety and depression. Also, and probably most profoundly, this means that we are far less likely to slip into the trauma response of fight/flight/freeze. We will look at this in more detail in the chapters on addiction and trauma.

Finding Strength

Yoga Saved My Life
Nancy Rose

Yoga set me free from self-hate and gave me a forever home.

I guess I'm what you call a recovering fake-happy/pleasure-seeking addict. An overall abuser of anything that brings superficial joy. Food, sex, alcohol, drugs. Addicted to validation and love from anything outside my being.

Feeling hostage to my life and my mind, like I had no control, no choice, I was either manipulative about getting what I wanted or so deeply miserable that I couldn't wait to start numbing that out with external relief.

Yoga was the first glimpse into self-sustaining my own happiness. I knew it was yoga that was going to be the path to finding my peace. I was not willing to feel like 'that' anymore.

Yoga set me free from that self-hate and introduced me to self-love. Connecting me to an understanding of radical self-acceptance and reaching for unconditional self-love every day. Ultimately, yoga reunited me with my intuition, which allowed for my own personal and spiritual realisation. I never have to look outside for love again. And for that I believe yoga saved my life.

His feet suck secret virtue of the Earth.
                                    Wilfrid Owen, 'The Wrestlers'

CHAPTER SEVEN

I'm Stuck

Yoga Saved My Life
Yelena Veliko

Watching my mother's mental illness progress meant seeing the mother I loved disappear.

My resilience became evident to me early in life. My mom was replaced by a stranger who spent most of her time in alternate realms.

At twenty-one, I lost her from my life completely, and consequently lost myself. I graduated college, found a job, a partner. But, despite appearances, a high-pitched ringing anxiety consumed me.

Eventually, this perfectly constructed, safe life started to erode. I was on the precipice of a remarkable opportunity for either growth or destruction. I chose the former – to confront my essence and create a new life as the best and truest version of myself.

Yoga called to me. For the first time in many years, I was intentionally focused on nourishing my soul, mind and body.

My practice has taught me to know, love and trust myself. I have learned countless lessons about the power of patience and persistence. I have found my centre for when I start to spin away.

I'm Stuck

> Most importantly, I am no longer a prisoner to that painful anxiety that riddled me for years. I have the strength to make decisions based on my dreams, not my fears.
>
> Yoga was the vehicle in my journey out of a mundane, directionless existence and into a purposeful, powerful, mindful and joyful life of perpetual growth.

Many of us feel that we will only be accepted if we conform to certain expectations – if we make ourselves speak and act in certain ways; ways that will make our parents love us, our friends like us, or our colleagues respect us – even if to do so means contorting ourselves into a square hole we know we are too round for. We get stuck in ways of being that don't really suit us, yet we are too scared to show the more authentic version of ourselves for fear of rejection. We become very clear about what is 'me' and what is 'not me'.

Many clients tell me 'I am/am not the sort of person who…' And my heart always sinks slightly when they do. I don't ever like to think that any of us are only one sort of person. I think that true health comes from having access to all aspects of ourselves – a full cast of characters on the stage, a full orchestra of instruments if you prefer an auditory analogy, or, if you are more visually minded, the entire spectrum of colours in our own rainbow. We can be woodwind one day and percussion the next, green one day, red the next, never just 'one sort' of a person. Yet so many of us feel we have got stuck in one identity – 'I am a strong person,' 'I am a weak person,' 'I am a leader,' 'I am a follower,' 'I'm artistic, beautiful, clever, practical, ugly, unlikeable, clumsy, introvert, extrovert…' The list of identities we get stuck in is endless and often determined at a very young age when we were desperate to define ourselves. Or had ourselves defined by others. This is very limiting and cuts us off from many essential constituents.

Unsticking

How can we get away from seeing ourselves as only one thing? In therapy we explore all the various forces, experiences and relationships that have made and shaped our one-sided view of ourselves. We can come to understand how ingrained traits have moulded us, and so look at them from different angles, uncovering the various lenses we have consequently developed through which we see the world, and therefore ourselves. Unconditional positive regard can make room for, and make it safe for, other characters to tentatively step out onto the stage without fear of ridicule and the paralysis that can bring.

Can yoga provide a similarly accepting response?

'Stuckness' is often mirrored in our bodies. We increasingly seize up as we get older, a physical representation of becoming more and more set in our ways, entrenched in one way of being. By practising yoga, you will become more flexible, physically and otherwise. Yoga will help you to break through your personal paralysing emotional and physical blocks; and, by now, you should hopefully know that there are ways you can do that kindly and gently.

Physiologically, yoga gets the juices flowing, mirroring what we need to be able to do with our minds. Nothing embodies this idea better than the constant movement of the spine through its full range of motion – forward, backward, sideways and twisting.

Moving the spine in all directions also shows us symbolically that we can be less stuck in one way of being, or in the feeling that we have only one way out.

Another advantage of yoga is how it leads the muscles to alternate between lengthening and contracting, thus encouraging them to find their full expression as well.

Movement also stimulates the production of synovial fluid, an egg-white-textured liquid found in the joints that can be likened to the oil in a car engine or on a bike chain preventing rust and seizure. It lubricates joints, reduces friction between them, acts as a shock absorber to protect a joint and its cartilage from wear and tear and stops the joints freezing up. It allows the bones to glide around fluidly. Symbolically, this greater ease of movement helps us to un-box ourselves from those corners into which we've retreated.

Synovial fluid also acts as a filter for keeping harmful cells out. Without enough synovial fluid, the joints can get inflamed – and this worsens with age and conditions like arthritis – all the more reason to take up or keep going with yoga as we age and start to get more stuck in our ways, viewpoints and bodies.

As therapy lets us 'try on for size' the unused parts of ourselves and find a voice for them, so yoga lets us physically embody different stances and shapes. And just as therapy helps us verbally and emotionally find new lenses through which to see ourselves, so can yoga via more literal, embodied means provide new ways of envisaging our place in the world.

We can alter our perspective – literally – by turning everything on its head and looking at the world from over our shoulders, through our legs or upside down. There are two groups of postures that particularly enable us to do that. Let's start turning our fixed ideas on their heads.

Inversions

Turning yourself upside down enables you to literally look at things from a new angle, and so invites a change of perspective – which may lead to a change in behaviour. It doesn't have to be a complicated or advanced posture. Yes, *sirsasana* (headstand), *adho mukha vrksasana* (handstand) and *urdhva dhanurasana* (wheel, a deep backbend) require great physical strength and agility. However, others are more accessible. For instance, *uttanasana* (standing forward fold) and *adho mukha svanasana* (downward dog) are often repeated over and over again in a class and regularly take you upside down. Downward dog takes your gaze not only upside down but also backwards, with a view through your own legs. It is disorientating, but that's the point. There are many ways of viewing the world and it can look – and feel – very different from each perspective.

Inversions place the head below the heart, an idea we came across earlier. Symbolically speaking, the heart being higher than the head invites us to ask – do we normally 'lead' with head or heart? Which do we let guide us? Which is more likely to have the answer we desire? Can we listen to the possibility that we could be who our hearts would really like us to be?

There are other benefits to inversions. Headstand and handstand are quite advanced postures, and each requires a great deal of strength balanced with flexibility. So already here you are having to call on two different skills, and few of us naturally possess high levels of both. Maybe you rely on your strength and brute force to haul your way through life. That won't work here; you need some flexibility to counteract it. Or are you maybe rather 'floppy', bending to the will of others and swaying with the prevailing tide? This flexibility alone is not going to help you get and stay upside down unless you can also access your inner, core strength.

And then there are all the potential falls you might encounter on the way up into your inversion, all of which will challenge your notion that you are good at this and can rely on what you know. Each and every fall will help you to learn patience, humour, how to address your fears and how to accept failure as a necessary part of success.

Inversions take you out of your comfort zone, force you not to do the same old, same old, not to rely on familiar skills and tricks. You really will need to feel the fear and do it anyway, thereby learning that the unfamiliar is possible and that once you get there, the view is different — more startling, more curious, more sparkling even, as you get to see the world anew.

Inversions also have great physiological benefits.

When you turn yourself upside down, the blood flow is sent in the opposite direction to normal, as is the flow of cerebral spinal fluid, and your lymphatic drainage is reversed. The overused feet get a much-needed break, while the brain gets an increased flow of blood; this means increased availability of oxygen and glucose, which makes it more able to produce the mood-boosting hormones dopamine and serotonin. And with better mood comes a greater ability to work with life's challenges.

Inversions increase the relaxation response, and heart rate, breathing rate and blood pressure all slow and lower.

Anatomically, inversions strengthen, extend and tone the postural muscles of the neck, torso and back: in fact, all the muscles needed to help us challenge gravity. Symbolically, gravity is constantly pulling us down (remember the slumped shoulders of depression), as are our ingrained ways of thinking. Ways of thinking that feel like unstoppable forces telling us we cannot fight the way we are meant to be. We think we cannot fight gravity – yet upside down here we are, challenging the status quo. Inversions strengthen us against that sink into inevitability – we can contest it. With effort and kindness and understanding, and with many falls en route, we can be who we want to be.

And by strengthening the neck, torso and limb girdle muscles we are helping to support our posture when we stand too; we will gain a straighter spine and a better-aligned head atop it – the perfect stance with which to face the fear of change.

As always with any of the yoga postures and techniques I mention, you need a good teacher instructing you how to do them safely. Inversions done badly can cause injury, so do not attempt them without help.

Twists

Like inversions, twisting postures really epitomise how a different viewpoint can open up a new field of possibility. Their fantastic ability to undo physical stuckness – moving us through another plane of motion – can help create that internal fluidity we all need if we are not to get stuck in one story.

Twists rotate and stretch the muscles of the back. They restore a motion that we tend to lose easily as we rarely perform this movement in everyday life. A twist bathes the vertebrae and joints in synovial fluid, keeps them buoyant and defying gravitational pull and helps prevent them shortening, hardening or getting fused. The surrounding muscles and soft tissue too all benefit from this movement to counteract our sedentary lifestyles.

The increase in mobility that twists encourage is particularly helpful for anyone with digestive issues. A sense of sluggishness in this area can be very symbolic of how stagnant we have become in other ways.

As with inversions, twists are also somewhat disorientating as they involve a crossing of the body's lateral line and a view over a different shoulder, with all the symbolism that involves. The brain has to again work a tiny bit harder to work out what we are looking at and what is going on. This opens up the mind to all sorts of possibilities.

Twists show us how from a place of stuckness, we can expand. The first instruction when going into any twist is to lengthen the spine, which physically gives us space between the vertebrae to then twist further, and symbolically reminds us both how far we can go, and also how much further we could go. It's a good lesson to learn – the tighter we are in our bodies and opinions, the less we can expand. If we have more freedom to move, if we are more flexible, we are more open, both literally and metaphorically.

Find Your *Drishti*

Drishti means 'focused gaze' and is an important concept in yoga. On a practical level, your *drishti* helps you concentrate, so can be particularly helpful to keep your balance when standing.

Symbolically, too, the idea of *drishti* relates strongly to both twists and inversions, both groups of postures that allow us to look in different directions to our norm.

When in an inversion or a twist your line of sight is disrupted. The familiar seems different, which means you become more aware of the sense of sight, and more curious about what you are looking at. When you are next upside down or twisted round, take a look at something in the room – your sofa or your rug, or a picture on the wall. You may notice that you need to look much more closely, and that you become much more focused on it as you look at it through this new lens. Disrupt your normal gaze and you may well learn more about the world and about yourself.

We have many idioms and phrases to do with sight, look and gaze, which shows how significant they are and how far they go beyond a purely literal meaning:

- second sight
- hindsight
- to lower or raise your sights
- to have the scales drop from your eyes
- to be blind to the truth
- to have a 'point of view' or a 'vision of the world'
- to keep your eyes on the prize

All of these and more point to the connection between our literal gaze and our deeper knowing.

Paying attention to our *drishti* teaches us to see the world more clearly and to develop concentrated attention. Where our eyes are directed, our attention follows.

Confining your visual focus to one point, literally when using a *drishti*, means your attention isn't dragged from pillar to post, helps you balance and encourages the mind to turn inwards.

I'm Stuck

Drishti is both a technique and a metaphor, training us to be less overwhelmed by our very visually stimulating external world. Turning it more towards the internal world helps develop *insight*. It helps render the invisible visible, just as in therapy we try to render the unconscious conscious, to examine it in the clear light of day where it can do less harm.

Yoga, and especially those postures which disorientate, can help shift things quite dramatically. If you alter your body, your sight and your aim, then your world view and your view of yourself will follow, making it all too obvious that you are not only one sort of person – you can be many, all of them fulfilling.

Whose Story Is This Anyway?

Having spent some time understanding the importance of recognising our own viewpoint, and discovering value in disrupting that perspective occasionally, now seems a good moment to look at the viewpoint of this book and its author – me.

Never forget that everything you read comes from a certain vantage point, is seen through a certain lens. I am writing this book via my own lens as a white, middle-class, middle-aged woman who lives in a busy Western city in the twenty-first century and inhabits three roles – writer, therapist and yoga teacher. I have read, studied and experienced a lot of different types of yoga and different types of psychotherapy, I have travelled widely, and I work hard at keeping an open mind and an awareness of my own positioning and subjectivity. Yet I have to acknowledge my starting point, and the fact that I am the only person who has experienced the unique set of events that have occurred in my life, each one of which has given me different experiences to each one of you.

This is true for all of us, and I am sharing these pages with a whole myriad of different voices from the wide Fierce Calm community, each also coming from their own unique perspective, and thereby enriching my own. Nevertheless, I control the narrative of this book and my own lens is my own lens. It is important for all of us to remain aware that someone is always controlling the narrative – of every book you read and of every class you take. Always remember that other narratives, other teachers, are available. There are many other lenses through which we could be exploring yoga, and psychotherapy, and the parallels between them. These are mine.

Yoga itself is an evolving process of shifting perspectives – it is verb, not noun. To talk about traditional or classical yoga throws up a whole raft of questions. Which tradition? Which era? Whose narrative is driving each version? History is not divorced from the culture in which we learn it. Many scholars are writing fascinating theses on these very questions and this is not the book in which to explore them, but it is important to know that the debate is raging and will continue to rage because nothing ever stands still. It cannot stand still because we evolve or we die. The world changes and we have to change with it and yoga has similarly adapted over the years, and over ever more diffuse areas of the globe, and via the different types of teachers who disseminate it. The only constant is change. And in the same way, Western psychotherapy has also diversified and taken different approaches in the quest for better mental, physical and emotional health and engagement with the self and the world.

All of this highlights why it is so important to value and trust your own experience – something that both therapy and yoga encourage you to do. The self-knowledge, self-awareness and resulting self-confidence you will gain means that you become your own best teacher and guide. You become able to question what you are told and see if it fits with what you know for yourself. Buddha told us that the finger pointing at the moon is not the moon. Try out your teachers' suggestions but know that your own subjective feedback – a feedback loop you are honing and refining with every yoga practice – is more useful than slavishly following their precise cues. They have not had your experiences and they do not inhabit your unique body.

Yelena says it so well when she describes yoga as her vehicle for perpetual growth. I too have found myself growing and learning and needing yoga to provide me with different things at different times in my life.

For instance, in my early twenties I had an incredibly busy job in the media and found Sivananda yoga gave me the permission I couldn't give to myself to take things slowly, spend time on each asana and also spend time in *savasana* (corpse pose) between each one. As my strength and resilience grew, and my interest in yoga along with them, I found I was drawn more to the yoga of B. K. S. Iyengar. The close attention to alignment, the discipline, the physical challenge; all these things were helpful in counteracting what had become the rather chaotic, and yes, still stressful life of a late-twenties, early-thirties person in the media, as I was then. After about a decade, I found this style and its discipline no longer fitted with what I needed. It was becoming apparent that Iyengar's strict instructions, based on his own male, Indian body type, were no longer really useful and I needed the freedom to explore more what my female, English, and now slightly older body type needed. This led me to Scaravelli yoga with its emphasis on connection with the Earth, close attention to the spine and honouring one's own experience. It gave me the space to explore what was right for me as I started to think about slowing down, finding a secure base and increasing flexibility alongside the strength. When I changed jobs at forty to become a psychotherapist and was no longer running around as much as I had in my media career, I found I wanted to up the pace yogically again, so I started alternating my Scaravelli classes with some more dynamic-flow classes. When I began teaching yoga I realised that all these very different influences were informing my teaching, allowing me to be more flexible and responsive both in how I taught and within my own practice.

Just as we adapt our clothing and our habits to each changing season, so we can adapt our yoga practices to suit where we are in our lives. But the one thing that will always be with you in any sort of practice is your body, so never lose touch with it and your changing needs. Teachers (and writers) are there to guide you, not to command you. They are but fingers pointing at the moon; it is up to you to find the moon for yourself.

When I let go of what I am, I become who I might be.
                                                                Lao Tzu

CHAPTER EIGHT

Going Into Battle

Yoga Saved My Life
Charlie Dark

For a young black boy growing up in pre-gentrified south London the art of puffing up your chest, learning to scowl and walking with a bop to appear harder than you could ever hope to be were skills perfected at an age when the white kids in my school were still playing with Action Man.

Racism taught me that in order to survive I had to become my own Action Man, my own superhero, the king of my own kingdom and that vulnerability was an emotion never to be displayed.

Couple this with a home environment where the expectations placed upon my shoulders were doubled by the hopes of a generation of immigrants' dreams and it was no surprise that depression and anxiety soon manifested in my brain.

My latest career left turn was done for self-preservation and a mission to take the mysterious world of yoga to the people who need it most.

It's a heavy stone to push up the hill yourself and the wellness industry knows it has a lack of diversity but thankfully, it's a problem that's slowly beginning to be addressed.

> While we wait for the industry to realise its duty in the healing process, let us close our eyes for two minutes and take the deepest of breaths. Breathe in goodness, breathe out the bad. Repeat times infinite until balance is restored. Bless up, people, and have an awesome day.

'What protects the child imprisons the adult.'

I don't know who came up with this, but I like how evocative it is. For me it conjures up an image of a frightened, confused child strapping on a suit of armour.

It can be frightening being a child and trying to understand what is expected of us. We have seen how strong is the need to conform, to not show the ways in which we are different. Sometimes we are even mocked for our sensitivities, which might get labelled as weaknesses. So we hide them deep inside where no one will be able to taunt or dislike us because of them. We put on this armour to protect ourselves from the wounds that inevitably come with feeling vulnerable or just a bit 'wrong', rendering us desperate to mould ourselves into the person we think our parents wish us to become or that our friends deem acceptable.

Who wouldn't want to create a handy suit of armour to deflect all the arrows of disapproval that might otherwise land and pierce the soft flesh of our tender underbellies? It's a sensible adaptation to a frightening world. Until it isn't. We grow up and need to adapt, but our armoured suit often stays the same size, trapping us inside what has now become a cage or prison. The armour is now far too small. It constricts our breathing, infringes our free movement and, most importantly, prevents us growing into the fully rounded adult, we can be.

This building of defences – both physical and emotional – was recognised very early on by Sigmund Freud. He, and others who later built on his work, identified several 'defences' that most of us employ to protect our vulnerable inner child. A very common, and perhaps the most obviously literal one is to fashion yourself a hard outer shell of 'strength', toughness, invincibility. These psychological defences often have a physical corollary and yoga provides the perfect vehicle for working with that.

Forms of Armour

We've already seen how our bodies can sometimes reveal our emotions very literally – the folded-in depressive, the floaty non-coper, the speediness of the anxious person. And Charlie describes so eloquently how he had to perfect the art of sticking out his chest as though it were a breastplate to deflect all criticism; scowling and walking with a bop, all to give the impression of 'hardness'. Others may stand with their legs wide and braced, muscles bulging, building barricades made of muscle tension, all while feeling like jelly inside.

As well as obvious forms like displays of physical strength and bravado, or a swaggering stance, our armour can be built of vast financial security; of political or corporate success and power; of global fame or infamy; of intellectual superiority and verbal dexterity.

Defences are necessary to protect us against hurt and pain. However, they can also 'protect' us against more pleasurable emotions – things like warmth, love, respect and joy, that can come with deeper connection, with a more honest communication of our vulnerabilities.

Can we find healthier, more authentic ways of managing those feelings of vulnerability? Can we feel less shame about having them in the first place? You won't be surprised to learn that, through yoga and psychotherapy, I think we can.

In a psychotherapeutic relationship we start by recognising the defences, slowly understanding the vulnerabilities they hide, and then gently exploring ways to accept these vulnerabilities, cradling, soothing and giving permission to the softness; finding ways to work with them that aren't so restrictive and don't make us feel so stuck with only one way of responding. But this can only happen in a deep and dependable relationship when a client feels safe enough and trusts that they won't be shamed for feeling this way.

Your yoga practice is similarly starting that process of building trust in yourself, as you learn compassionate self-awareness that lets your bodymind know you are listening and not going to harm it. With trust established, your practice can then assist you in recognising, dissolving and refashioning your protective mechanisms. You can come to understand your own embodied expression of all the same phenomena we've been discussing – whether that be the crab-like, rounded back of depression, the inflated chest of anger, the tensed jaw of stress or whatever other habits are slowly being revealed by your growing yogic awareness. By showing commitment to your practice, by setting aside time to do it and by learning to listen to your body compassionately, you have already begun this process. Your body will have started to understand that you will listen and treat it carefully and respectfully. This, and the other grounding practices we have seen so far, have created a bedrock, a 'secure base' for the trusted relationship you need for your body to feel safe enough to soften. As it does, it will gradually show you where and how it has been armouring its most tender parts.

As always, it is a well-rounded yoga practice that can help to eventually dissolve those imprisoning suits of armour that you have outgrown, and help you to realise your real inner strength – a strength that comes from working with the vulnerabilities instead of burying them; a strength that comes from grounding yourself and finding that secure place.

One category of postures that help soften the armour and allow access to the deeper emotions is the hip openers, and other poses that focus on the pelvic area.

Don't be surprised if the tears start to flow as you allow long-held wounds to reopen and heal. This has happened to me, and I've seen it happen to many others in my classes – bursting into tears as emotions we didn't know we had find expression.

- **Opening the pelvic area**

Our metaphorical mask of invincibility is reflected in our muscle patterns and ways of holding. And nowhere is this truer than in the tender underbelly, home to precious internal organs, and the seat of our sense of self. Consequently, a lot of emotion gets stored within the pelvic area and the hips.

The hip joint is the largest joint in the body and some of the most powerful muscles extend across it (notably the psoas). It is crucial for providing stability and support. It enables us to:

- keep the spine upright so we're ready to meet challenges
- take charge, by giving us the ability to walk towards or away from what is beneficial or harmful
- run from danger
- curl into the foetal position when attacked

So this area is fundamental to our most basic needs and instincts for survival. Because of this, and the need to protect the tender organs lying deep within the pelvis's protective casing, this is an area we tend to clench, tighten, grip and brace against fear, hardening it – locking the armour into place.

It is therefore important, but not easy, to learn to soften here. There are many, many poses you can choose to help you open and render more pliable this delicate area. There are gentle limbering warm-ups, the supine *supta baddha konasana* (reclining bound angle or cobbler), the seated *sukhasana* (easy pose – that's its translation, not necessarily what you will experience it as!) or the more energetic *natarajasana* (dancer). Different poses will feel more appropriate for your intention and energy on any given day.

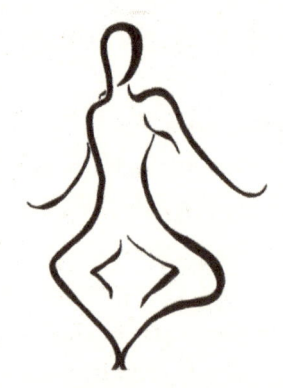

Supta Baddha Konasana

Key to these postures is taking the time to work your way into them and then staying with them, breathing into the area, sending loving thoughts there and paying close attention to where the tightness lies and to any emotions that start to manifest.

Just as hip opening gives us greater range of motion, making the other postures easier to do, so emotional opening gives us a greater range of e-motion. By which I mean that being more open to the world inside and out gains access to that full spectrum of colour, that fully rounded, full cast of characters. And it opens us up to other people more as well. It's a bit like saying you show me yours – your vulnerability – and I'll show you mine. This leads to much deeper connection with others. When you find compassion for your own softer sides, you will find more compassion for those of other people too, and invite their compassion for yours.

- **Stretch the psoas**

The psoas muscle attaches to your spinal column before passing deeply through the pelvis to join the top of the femur (thighbone), connecting your trunk to your legs. Its deeply buried location means that in metaphorical terms it stores some of your most deeply hidden emotions and secrets.

Being a deep muscle, it is not the easiest to access; but it is important, both to help get into the emotional holding associated with the hips in general and also because it acts as a bridge between the upper and lower halves of the body.

A tight psoas hampers free movement of the limbs and pelvis; so releasing the psoas brings greater freedom of movement that enables torso and lower limbs to work in better harmony. Removing blockages on this essential bridge enables the free passage of fluids throughout the body, helps release the diaphragm and so supports the internal organs above, as well as providing a sensation of grounding and centring below. These are all physical effects that aid the sense of safety and containment needed to access our emotional wounds. Metaphorically, if you feel that your options have become limited, that your vitality has decreased, you lack core awareness or connection to the inner sensations that are so necessary to understanding our internal selves, rediscovering these connections will help you to find greater trust in your own instincts.

Postures such as pigeon pose (*eka pada rajakapotasana*) and lunges can help bring feeling to this hard to access region.

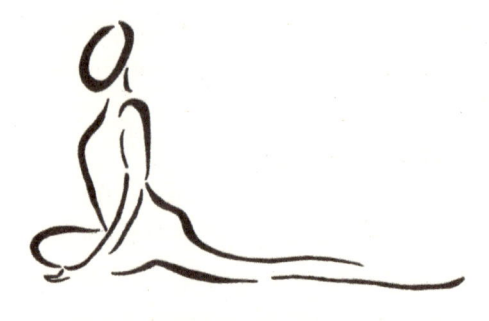

Eka Pada Rajakapotasana

- **Counterbalancing for protection**

As we saw earlier on, generally we learn very young – often while we are pre-verbal – to shut away the softer, more secret parts of ourselves. Reopening them therefore puts us back in touch with younger parts or versions of ourselves – hence the weeping that often results. While liberating and cathartic, this can also be frightening and disorientating. I cannot say often enough that you need to work gently and compassionately here.

We might use our time in therapy to talk to, connect with, the inner child, give them their long-denied voice. In yoga we can connect to them through movement and awareness. This delicate child needs to know they are no longer alone; that there is a grown-up version of you who can take care of their fears. But part of that care-taking involves knowing when to put some armour – a better-fitting, more comfortable version – back in place. Therapeutically, that might mean gaining an understanding of which people or situations are not safe for your vulnerable selves and knowing that in these circumstances it is okay to call on the tougher parts of you to take the lead – but doing so in the full knowledge that you are accessing the 'tough guy' character for a reason; it's not who you have to be all the time.

In your yoga practice, part of building safety and trust comes from letting your body know that while you may take it somewhere it didn't initially want to go, you will always make sure it can return to the place of safety it knows. In Chapter Ten we will go into more depth about counterbalancing – it is an important yoga skill whatever postures you've been doing – and with hip opening, when we have really let it all out and exposed ourselves, it is especially important.

Think about, and feel into, what you might need to do to make yourself less vulnerable before returning to the real world. Maybe you need to do the closed-hip *virabhadrasana* 1 if you've been doing the open-hipped *virabhadrasana* 2. Maybe you could do *garudasana* (eagle) if you've been lying in *supta baddha konasana* (reclining bound angle). Or if the whole practice has left you feeling exposed, then what about resting in folded over *balasana* (child) instead of spreading yourself open in *savasana*?

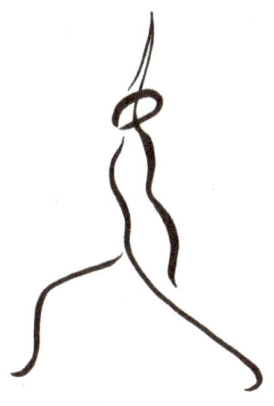

Virabhadrasana 1

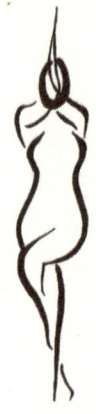

Garudasana

Experiencing more range and openness in the hip area, opening yourself to emotion and authenticity, can give you an experience of, and offer access to, parts of yourself you may never have known existed, revealing a greater range of possibility in other areas of your life. As you open your hips and other closed-off areas, you allow that fuller rainbow of colours to expand and shine more brightly. You start to feel what access to the full complement of selves that lie within you might offer.

> *Nothing is softer or more flexible than water, yet nothing can resist it.*
>
> Lao Tzu

CHAPTER NINE

I Feel Vulnerable

Yoga Saved My Life
Donna Noble

Becoming ill with Bell's palsy (where one side of the face becomes paralysed) was when I began to re-evaluate my life. Initially I was embarrassed by this very visible illness, and hid away – only going to places where my friends would accept me.

After five years of living with the condition and trying everything advised by the medical profession there was no improvement and I accepted it. It was as though I had given up.

The illness turned out to be a gift to help me change my life. I often ask the question – if I had my life over, would I eliminate the Bell's? I don't think I would: it has defined me in ways I could not have imagined.

I have become passionate about body image. I realised that my body is a miracle – not something to be taken for granted.

Working in the corporate world, life was stressful and my work/life balance was out of sync. I conformed to every expectation society tells us makes us happy: house, car, career. But I was disconnected from the 'real' me – carefree, spontaneous.

> Eventually, I was made redundant: the best thing that happened to me, forcing me to change.
>
> The choice to teach came from a deeper sense of knowing – from my gut.
>
> This thing called yoga was organically carving out another path for me that felt so right.
>
> The change starts within you and then you will be able to change the world in whatever way you were meant to.

We've talked about the masks we wear, the selves we allow out, the armour we strap on, the defences we construct. All these strategies have one aim – to hide what we perceive as weakness. But sometimes we experience the opposite problem – our armour feels too heavy to pick up, let alone get inside. We find ourselves showing our helplessness all too often, feeling naked, exposed and fearful.

And that can bring up a lot of shame. We feel less than, or incapable, or a failure. Sometimes we feel completely defeated, as if we have nothing left with which to prop ourselves up. We've run out of resources. If it lasts long enough we can get stuck in a 'victim' role, thinking we are hopeless and unable to change, looking for others to save us, searching for the answer externally as opposed to where it really matters – internally.

We can even start to identify with this image of ourselves, to the point that we assume we can't change or that we really are 'weak'. Chances are, none of those things is true and we just need to find our inner strength, as opposed to allowing society to define us by what we can't do.

I Feel Vulnerable

Yoga can help you find your inner strength, teach you how much you are able to withstand, help you see that it is often far more than you thought. And nothing is more symbolically representative of strength than the warrior poses.

- **Warrior poses**

These pretty much do what they say on the tin. They evoke our inner warrior, that part that we all possess but sometimes lose touch with; the part prepared to stand its ground and stand up for what it believes in.

Notice how my two last phrases both use the word 'stand', and how common, and how useful this word is when we are trying to describe what inner conviction feels like. (Look at page 114 to see just how often the word crops up in common phrases and idioms around the idea of groundedness, stability and fortitude.)

Standing poses in general enable us to embody and feel into the power of that sensation physically, putting us in touch with this quality of rock-like integrity.

The warrior poses give us a particularly strong embodied sense of what it can feel like to really stand up for oneself, and of how empowering that can be. These poses activate those elements needed to viscerally feel our strength – the solid, fortified base that comes from strong, stable legs; the inner core of fire that comes from drawing energy inwards to energise us; and the focused aim and reach that literally and metaphorically keeps our sights fixed on our goal.

It might seem strange that such a compassionate practice as yoga uses images of warriors, who more usually evoke thoughts of conflict and battles. But *virabhadra*, the Sanskit word, breaks down into:

vira = hero
bhadra = companion or friend

Put the two together and you get a sense of an awe-inspiring companion whose role is to help and protect, not fight. Someone who stands for (there it is again) loyalty and bravery. And of course, we are ultimately learning to be that person for ourselves. This is one of the reasons why I like to use the Sanskrit. Knowing the etymology can reveal a lot, such as not so much 'doing' a posture as embodying it, feeling into what it means to become the quality it is representing – in this case combining courage with compassion.

In all of the warrior poses the lower body provides a solid, strong foundation, our pillar of support. Muscularly we are strengthening and toning the large muscles of the legs, particularly the thighs, as well as in the ankles and feet. We have already come to understand the importance of creating a solid base, and how that base begins with a grounded connection to the feet, and through them to the Earth. We tune in to this as a strong *virabhadrasana* starts, as do all standing poses, by finding that connection to the Earth and rooting ourselves through steady, stable feet.

Grounded and safe within this firm base, weight equally distributed between both feet, we increasingly build that physical strength in the feet, ankles and legs. On and off the mat, we thereby gain confidence that nothing can push us off course (remember the Weeble!). As our physical strength increases so too does our inner strength, bolstered by the need to focus our gaze while holding this pose. This calm, steady gaze — the *drishti* — encourages us here in the moment, and in our wider life, to dwell and make decisions from a calm place of clarity, providing a true, steady, grounded aim.

In psychotherapy, attachment theory showed us that a firm base makes us feel more secure in ourselves, enabling us to explore and reach out for what we want in life. In the warrior poses we can

I Feel Vulnerable

physically experience how the solid, downward pull of the lower body acts to liberate the upper body, enabling it to reach freely and expansively towards our goal. Think about a tree trunk – it's the depth of the roots and the strength of the trunk that allow the branches to grow towards the sky and bear fruit and leaves.

The connection between the two halves of the body is the torso. In the warrior postures the torso, and all within it, is called on to be engaged and alive; the abdomen is slightly drawn in to activate and use the strength of the core and the heart is open and willing. The hips are flexible and unlocked. In all three *virabhadrasana* variations the whole body is working as a team, fluidly and in equilibrium.

In *virabhadrasana* 1, the forward-facing version, the arms are up, shooting towards the sky, visually and viscerally representing how high you can travel, how inspired you can be, how unlimited your reach – if rooted in a solid base.

In *virabhadrasana* 2 the body faces sideways, yet the eyes face forwards, towards your goal. One arm reaches out, steadily, arrow-like towards a target; the other reaching behind. You are neither leaning forwards into the future, nor leaning back into the past; you are upright, centred right in the middle, in the here and now, stable and immovable and ready to face whatever is coming at you.

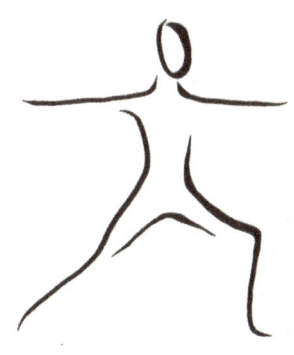

Virabhadrasana 2

Virabhadrasana 3 sees you on one leg, arms reaching dynamically forwards, towards your aim. It is more complex physically, both in terms of the muscle strength needed to hold you there and the concentration to stay balancing on one leg. However, when fully embodying and enjoying it, you will believe you can fly – and this gives you a sense of your power and all that is possible for you if you are steady and focused, your entire bodymind working together and concentrated on your aim, ready to launch.

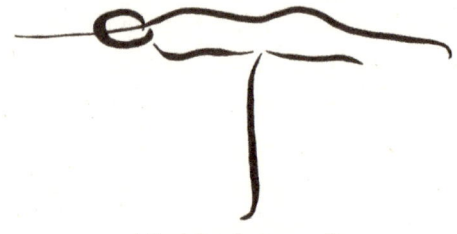

Virabhadrasana 3

All of the warrior poses cultivate strength, stability, determination and a readiness to embrace whatever comes at you, to deal with it in the present and in an open manner. They bring freedom, not from fear – that's impossible – but freedom from the thought that you cannot cope with it. So rather than fight fear, with the armour from the previous chapter, or flee it, giving up and accepting helplessness, they offer a third possibility – that maybe we can withstand fear bravely.

Maybe even more so if we couple them with our next series of postures – the arm balances.

• Arm balances
These postures, while not so symbolically obvious as the warriors, are fantastic for physically strengthening the upper body and arms. They tone and fortify these areas – with all the attendant emotional

I Feel Vulnerable

and figurative repercussions of increasing strength and confidence – in the same way that the warriors do for the lower body.

This creates the much-needed balancing out that I keep referring to. But it is also necessary for us to feel that we can protect this fragile area, home as it is to yet more delicate organs – the lungs and the heart.

Similarly to *virabhadrasana* 3, arm balances provide a solid, powerful connection to the Earth while leaving the legs light enough to feel they can fly. You start to believe you really are invincible.

Some of this comes from the realisation that more than just brute strength is required; the ability to lift comes only when it is coupled with the ability to simultaneously soften inside. An arm balance such as *bakasana* (crow) requires us to draw our tummies and thoughts inwards, knit into the core, find the focus and steadiness of our inner resolve, all while building up the necessary strength in the muscles of the arms. It's also about relaxing the joints and muscles, as opposed to hardening them. If you are to hold an arm balance, they need to release, not grip, and for that you need your groin, hamstrings, hips, knees and torso all to be as pliant and supple as possible. Perhaps counterintuitively, given how hard they look, it is a friendly, open and relaxed approach that will get you there, not rigid muscle-holding. This is also true for negotiating our way through our relationships.

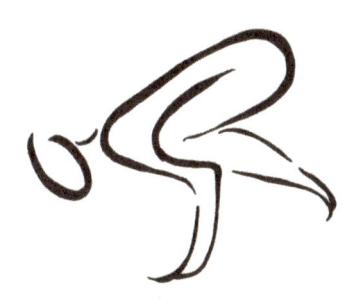

Bakasana

If you watch how naturally a child throws themselves upside down – into a handstand for instance – you will see how most of us, as adults, have lost the ability to not be scared of falling. It is this fear that stops us trying new things – whether that be a handstand or going for a promotion at work. Learning arm balances, with all the inevitable falls that will come along the way, can help us lose some of the fear and so regain some of the carefree freedom and sense of possibility we may have felt as children ourselves.

- **Balance strength with flexibility**

We've already seen that strength alone – just donning armour and going into battle mode – isn't always helpful. But also that losing our armour altogether and rendering ourselves helpless can be detrimental to our mental health. As in life, as in yoga.

Muscular strength won't help us if it is not balanced with flexibility; we need to rebuild our defences in a more helpful way, more relevant to how we are now.

In the film *Iron Man*, the protagonist's first attempt at a suit is rigid and solid and protects him but leaves no room for movement. With work, he comes up with one that is more sophisticated, more adapted to his actual body shape, more fluid and better fitting; it moves with him, adapts to each situation, rather than hampering him.

With yoga, we can move on from any stiff, outdated patterns of movement, ways of thinking or behaviours from our past and build ourselves a new pliable, adaptable and – most importantly – unique 'suit' that frees us to be who we are but doesn't leave us vulnerable.

Rigidity, hardness, external appearances: all will crumble if put under enough stress. Structures, people and concepts that incorporate flexibility and give can all withstand so much more. Rigidity

I Feel Vulnerable

is not at all conducive to change, makes us weaker in fact. Trees bend in the wind, and so survive; if they tried to remain rigid and upright they would snap and die after one storm.

In engineering, too, flexibility is key to strength; essential to any system that needs to adapt to internal or external changes.

Making sure we are primed to respond easily to change and uncertainty is surely one of the most useful things we can learn.

What yoga helps to develop is a more solid connection with yourself. A move away from what the influential psychotherapist Donald Winnicott called 'the false self'[17] and towards the often very frightened and hidden 'true self' (or more realistically, I believe, true 'selves', plural) sheltering within. When you can connect to more authentic versions of yourself you will no longer feel the need to play the victim, nor to rely on others to 'save you'. Their opinions will matter less, your own will matter more and this 'internal locus of evaluation', as we say in therapy, will be what guides you.

Let yoga help you find your inner warrior and learn to stand strong and proud in your own skin. It will reveal your true strength, as opposed to the fake bolstering of the armour, proving that strength comes *because* of your vulnerabilities, not despite them. No yoga pose will 'work' or endure if it relies purely on the brute force of either muscles or will and is not balanced by softness and fluidity.

Use your yoga postures to help you find that sweet spot where strength and flexibility meet without rigidity, where pliability and softness don't need to mean you are a pushover. In yoga and in therapy we recognise how important it is to not get trapped within such limiting binaries as 'I'm strong' or 'I'm weak'. We can – and need to – be both.

In the next chapter we will look more closely at why these polarities are so unhelpful and we will seek a way out of the prison they create.

Stand

Here are just some of the ways in which we connect the word 'stand' to the notion of strength, conviction and fortitude:

Stand for
Take a stand against
Stand by
Stand fast
Withstand
Take a firm stand
Stand up for
Stand on my own two feet
A house divided against itself cannot stand
Stand my ground
Know where I stand
An empty sack cannot stand upright
From my standpoint
It stands to reason
Stand up and be counted
A person who stands for nothing will fall for everything.

I Feel Vulnerable

Yoga Saved My Life
Greg Pember

At a young age I developed an intense obsession with creating a persona that would win others' approval.

In a fiercely competitive field of work I became a perfection addict. It was a fear-driven behavioural pattern that projected the 'Greg' that I thought people wanted to see, because if they saw who I really was – the real, messy and imperfect Greg – they would not work with me, or love and accept me.

I found myself in a downward vortex of fear and doubt. It was exhausting.

Yoga shifted everything. Yoga philosophy says that we already are the gift that this universe needs, with all our scars, imperfections and past wounds. Yoga offered me the framework to do the work I needed to use my old scars to empower myself.

I now practise letting myself be vulnerable, asking for what I need without my protective fear telling me that this will make me unloveable.

I can feel the love of the universe and the universal life force energy flow through me when I'm on my mat.

Through being intimate with my breath and the simplicity of the present moment I can hear the call to see myself as the universe already sees me: perfect, whole and complete. This is the invitation of yoga.

Not everything that is faced can be changed, but nothing can be changed until it is faced.

James Baldwin

CHAPTER TEN

The Swing of the Pendulum

Yoga Saved My Life
Finlay Wilson (Kilted Yogi)

My struggle with mental health is an ongoing thing that I experience every day. It isn't finished, and it probably won't be finished.

I tried to kill myself when I was eighteen. I had been in a secret same-sex relationship and when that ended, I got thrown back into the closet but it felt like a prison. I felt like a liar. I could see all the faces I lied to and my faith was tearing me to pieces. Obviously I didn't go through with it. But I did start exercising for the first time ever.

My path eventually led me to yoga. Yoga didn't fix anything.

But it has given me tools.

Something that would have thrown me off the precipice in the past now just stirs a little. The dark depths of my moods are less extreme. The whispers are still there. It's like a demon behind me waiting for me to be in pain enough, exhausted enough or beaten down enough. It's a seductive siren song.

The Swing of the Pendulum

So much of life is divided into binaries – good versus bad, right versus wrong. Or, as we saw in the last two chapters, strong versus weak, victim versus perpetrator. We've seen how limiting those identities can become if we get stuck at either pole, even if it can be useful to access both ends of the pendulum when the occasion demands.

Yoga, as we have seen over and over again, is all about the balancing of opposites. As Finlay says, it gives us tools to manage those swings, those extremes.

Balance in all its permutations – literal and metaphorical, physical and emotional – is the essence of yoga. And it is crucial to our mental health. Discovering balance, or equanimity, is one of the main reasons why yoga saves lives. Yoga will always draw our attention to when we have gone to one extreme or the other and bring us back to the centre, our secure base.

Think of how a tennis player, after a run to either edge of the court, always strives to return to the centre line, weight evenly balanced between each foot. If they are caught at the borderline they are forced to respond with any stroke they can make, weight more often than not forced onto one foot. And that is if they can even get to the ball at all. But from the centre line they have only half the distance to run for the next ball, their weight is centred so they can easily go in either direction and they have the choice to use any shot. They have given themselves options.

We too – in life and on the yoga mat – need to be able to get ourselves back to the middle.

Journeys to the Edge

You'll perhaps have noticed that I try very hard never to talk about absolutes, to say things are good or bad, or to use the words 'always' or 'never'. Very few behaviours are good or bad in and of themselves.

Instead, they may be more or less helpful for a given situation. Yet so often in life we stick to one or other of the extremes. We think we can only be strong, or a leader, or selfless, or 'on the go', because we are so afraid of the other polarity – being weak, or a follower, selfish or lazy. But there is a whole spectrum of possibility between the two sides.

In my therapy room, I see many people who have fixed notions of the best way to be. They dress up what is actually rigidity with words like strength, success, achievement, independence. They are terrified that if they give themselves an inch they will embark on a slippery slope to 'weakness' and 'failure', completely missing the point that true success, strength and achievement come from the open middle of the tennis court; from having the pliability and flexibility to span the entire spectrum, even if it might throw up difficulties along the journey. Remember Greg telling us in his story that he uses his scars to empower him (see page 115)?

In yoga classes I also see many people working from one or other end of the spectrum. There are students who love the activity and fear the stillness, or vice versa. Or those who love the extroversion of the backbends and resist or dread the introversion of the forward bends. We all need both, yet we all tend to find our place 'on the court' and stay there, cutting ourselves off from options that may be more helpful and, in the long run, make life easier.

We do want to be able to run for the edge of the court when necessary, but we also need to know how to return from it; we need the power that comes from being balanced in the centre.

Counterbalancing

Melanie Klein was a groundbreaking therapist working in the mid-twentieth century. Like John Bowlby, she understood the importance of the parent–infant relationship in shaping our view of ourselves. She identified the powerful internal pull we all have, from infancy, towards what she labelled 'splitting'[18] – wanting to see things as either all good or all bad. She saw the need for integrating these splits – in my metaphor, finding the middle of the court – as a developmental stage that we need to pass through, but she believed that, as with so much of our childhoods, we often don't get that chance. This is where therapy and yoga can help us, as adults, to experience a more nurturing relationship that can make amends for the earlier lack, and allow us to finally absorb these lessons.

Good yoga sequencing will take you to and fro between extremes – forwards to backwards, reaching up for the sky and reaching down into the Earth, hip closers after hip openers, for instance – in order to find the opposing force, and to counteract its effects. This counterbalancing means we are less 'split'. We have the ability to reach for either extreme – run to either side of the court – when we need to, but we don't need to get stuck there. We learn that we cannot only inhale, we need to exhale too. We cannot only ever forward bend, we also need to backbend.

In physical terms, you could say that the spine represents our balanced centre. It joins the head with the body, or, more symbolically, heaven with Earth, so representing connection. It also reveals the ordering, organising principle behind the polarities of forward and back, left and right and so on, and holds them together in a harmoniously functioning whole. The spine's symmetry allows you to observe imbalances – how the left side of the body feels as opposed to the right, the front as opposed to the back – become more aware of them, adjust, and so find better balance.

As always, there are certain elements of yoga that can be used to most effectively highlight the principle of balancing out extremes. The first one, ironically, is to feel what being unbalanced is like.

- **Take yourself off balance**

This exercise may seem simple but it is actually rather profound.

- Stand in *tadasana* (mountain) and close your eyes.
- Rock all your weight forwards into the balls of both feet, until you feel a faceplant coming on, then rock your weight back into your heels, until it feels like you are going to go over backwards.
- Sway to and fro and between these two extremes a few times, then make the motion smaller and smaller until you are making only micromovements between the two.
- Finally, come to stillness dead centre.
- Now take all your weight into your right foot, till your left becomes so light it could lift from the floor. Then do the same to the left. Again, sway to and fro a few times before finding your natural stillness dead centre.

You get the symbolic point, I'm sure. More importantly, you have embodied and felt it, physically.

You can apply this principle and action to almost any posture. In *virabhadrasana 2*, for example, your torso should sit lightly and upright midway between your widely spaced feet. To find what this balanced midpoint feels like, consciously reach your front arm to the front then the back arm to the back in a surfing motion and feel the inner effects. After a few reaches in both directions you will be able to feel your balanced middle much more easily.

- ***Dandasana***

This is staff, or rod pose and is an example of a very centred and balanced pose. It strengthens and aligns the spine – which here is upright, firm and grounded – and symbolises steadfastness. But

The Swing of the Pendulum

the arms and legs are crucial here too. If they lose focus, straightness or anchoring, the spine will, in turn, feel less strong and sure. The body works as its most harmonious whole only if each 'opposite' is given equal attention.

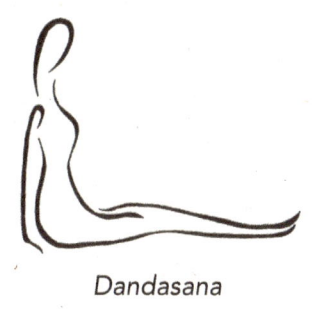

Dandasana

From this even, balanced pose, a relatively simple movement, albeit one requiring quite a bit of strength, lifts you into *purvottanasana* (upward plank). This posture opens and stretches the entire length of the front body. *Purva* means 'east', with all the connotations that brings – the rising of the sun, the dawning of our inner light, new beginnings, a surge in energy, burgeoning potential – and like all front-opening postures, *purvottanasana* is said to help us access the conscious mind and the future.

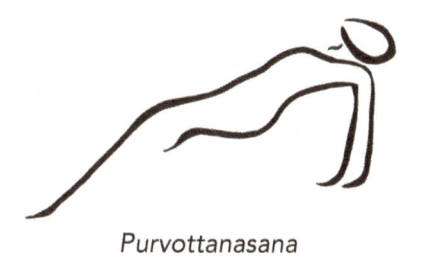

Purvottanasana

Contrast this with another relatively simple transition from *dandasana*, this one requiring more flexibility than strength, and going in the opposite direction – folding forwards into *paschimottanasana* (seated forward bend). *Paschima* means 'west' and this posture stretches the back of the body – said to be home to the unconscious mind, and our pasts. Folding forwards requires a softening, a surrender, and allows us to access the inner world of calm and recalibration.

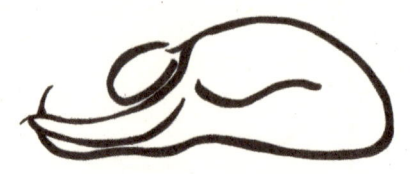

Paschimottanasana

So *dandasana*, in and of itself, represents and aids balance, and at the same time can act as the central safe space from which we can travel upwards and outwards, or downwards and inwards.

• Do sun salutations

Surya namaskar – the sun salutation – is a staple of many yoga classes. Why is it so useful and ubiquitous? It's because its flowing sequence of postures – to and fro, up and down, side to side – takes the body through a very wide range of motion, which is useful as a way of warming and waking up the body before launching into more complex or challenging postures.

It also neatly moves us from asymmetry to symmetry, from rest to activity, from an internal focus to an external. We go to the extreme of each in order to rediscover the balanced centre.

Doing sun salutations thus teaches that we cannot rely only on the familiar, on what we perceive to be the things we are good at. If we tend to rely on only our strength in life, a sun salutation shows that this needs balancing with flexibility. If we rely on flexibility alone, we discover in these movements the counteracting need for strength. A good analogy comes, perhaps, from looking at how our muscles work in pairs. Put very simply, in order to move a joint, one muscle – the agonist – must contract while its partner, the antagonist, must lengthen. And to lengthen it must relax. This push–pull collaboration between the pairs is what brings about movement, just as the push–pull between your contrasting selves will allow you to respond flexibly to different life situations.

These ideas of opposites and the need for counterbalance, and for integration of both extremes, is analogous to what Carl Jung would call our shadow side,[19] or what other approaches might call our less welcome 'selves' – those parts of ourselves we would rather not acknowledge but which, in fact, render us all the poorer for their lack.

Therapy and counterbalancing

The shadow self is something that comes up a lot in psychotherapy as we all tend to get stuck in rather literal versions of our polarities, terrified of allowing our shadow versions, the flipside of our characteristics, to get a look in. Let's take as an example those at the extreme where they see themselves as 'strong', are completely rigid in their defences and think any sort of flexibility is weakness. Such people often appear to be able to 'cope' because they analyse cognitively and ignore and override any emotion – they approach things top-down. They are often completely unaware that they even have a body, let alone listen to its messages – that's just too frightening because it might mean an emotion surfaces. This is often reflected by a physical tightness or reliance on muscular strength. People in this position need a therapist's help to access their feelings and their bodies, and a yoga practice to help them soften the clenched gripping.

At the other end of this scale are those who perhaps see themselves as failing or are completely swamped by their feelings. They cry and emote freely and can come across as chaotic and incapable – they approach things bottom-up. Physically, they may be overly flexible. The psychotherapeutic work with clients like this is to help them find their inner analytic resources and more cognitive abilities, while their yoga practice needs to focus more on grounding and building strength.

The Not Knowing

In both yoga and therapy we work on allowing ourselves access to both ends of the scale, on being able to explore both the shadow and the light. We work on softening the rigid, learning to yield in order to find flexibility in body and in attitude. And for the overly chaotic or collapsed we work towards finding strength, agency and empowerment.

All this can help us move towards understanding two of the hardest lessons to take on board, in therapy and in life:

- The need to hold in mind two opposing truths simultaneously: that sadness can be found alongside joy, gratitude in hardship, gems from within rubble, strength from pain.
- And the need to be okay with what can feel like a murky grey area in between certainties.

Can you be comfortable with not knowing? For it is here that we will find freedom; or, as Japanese essayist D. T. Suzuki put it: 'The mind that does not understand is the Buddha.'[20]

Yoga Saved My Life
Selena Garefino

My world has ended many times and been remade, with yoga the only constant.

So where do I start? Do I start with how yoga pulled me from my days as a homeless, eighth-grade dropout abusing drugs? Or do I tell you about how yoga gave me a home in my body when I was modelling at seventeen and being taught to loathe myself and my imperfections?

Should I begin with how my practice kept me from falling apart when I was living in the African bush caring for the dying? Or perhaps it saved my life more profoundly when it gave me a home inside myself once again in my own temple of flesh and bone after two major abdominal surgeries that literally gutted me.

Maybe the place to begin is how my practice gave me steadiness and kept me from falling into an irrevocable grief after I lost my spouse four weeks after we were married to severe brain trauma that left him violent and lost to me for ever.

This is how yoga has saved me. It has given me the tender resolve to not only withstand innumerable tragedies, but to rise strong and in love.

Praise and blame, gain and loss, pleasure and sorrow come and go like the wind.
To be happy, rest like a giant tree in the midst of them all.
The Buddha

CHAPTER ELEVEN

Spinning Out of Control

> ### Yoga Saved My Life
> **Jenny Clise**
>
> Yoga became my rock when I suffered from anxiety and panic. Anxiety has always been something I have struggled with, and yoga is something that empowers me to face all the things that cause me fear, anxiety, stress, etc. Yoga helps me work through each of them, by first acknowledging them. It is what makes me more content with the world around me, and confident in my ability to tackle all that life throws at me! I am lucky to have found yoga early in life. I wish I could tell people that mindful breathing can be just as powerful as any drug. I want more people to feel at home in their own bodies and minds, just as yoga has helped me to find home wherever I am.

Does life sometimes feel unmanageable in all sorts of ways? Outer chaos can so often be a representation of inner chaos. We've seen how through yoga we can unstick from being just one 'sort of person'. But giving up an 'identity', even one that was restrictive, can disorientate your sense of knowing who you are. It can feel discombobulating to be left in the liminal space between the old you that you would like

Spinning Out of Control

to cast off and the new you who you may not have yet found – as you transition towards integrating the many 'yous' you are and can be.

Perhaps you know that feeling of chaos and uncertainty? Of being out of control, perhaps lurching from crisis to crisis, out of touch with who you are and how you feel? Living life as though you are merely the passenger in a speeding car?

Yoga can help put you back in the driving seat. And that starts with noticing and acknowledging the vehicle in which you are a helpless passenger; recognising the state you are in and the state your body is in; accepting that where you are is where you are.

There's an old joke about someone asking directions and being told, 'Well, I wouldn't start from here.' But you do need to start from here. There really is no other way.

Yoga makes you come face to face with your 'here' like no other practice. Done mindfully and with awareness, it leaves nowhere to hide. This is a good (if perhaps initially daunting) thing. You have no choice but to accept where here is; and that's when the real choices open up. Rather than just firefighting, reacting to the slings and arrows of a chaotic life, you have agency and the confidence not only to know where 'there' is but also how to get yourself there.

We will look more at choice later, but for now let's take our own advice and start with here, today. And today's suggestions are more about attitude than they are about action.

We can learn a lot about attitude from another Eastern tradition that has – mercifully for us – also made its way to the West.

Beginner's Mind

Monk Shunryū Suzuki is widely credited with having brought Zen Buddhism to the West. His teachings on 'beginner's mind'

– *shoshin* – tell us that if we drop our preconceptions and expectations, empty our minds of all we think we know, we create space for new perceptions and viewpoints. In his seminal book, *Zen Mind, Beginner's Mind*, Suzuki explains how if your mind is empty, it is always ready for anything, it is open to everything. A beginner's mind holds many possibilities while the expert's has few.

You too can come to the yoga mat each time as though it is the first time. Don't project forwards to the things you feel you ought to be able to do, then get cross because you can't do them yet. Don't look back to what you did yesterday and assume that because you've done it once you can do it again. Just tune in. Listen to what your body is telling you is needed and possible today.

This mirrors what we do in psychotherapy. We try to accompany our clients into the present moment, helping them feel safe enough to inhabit who they are, not who they expect themselves to be, or have always been. We help bring them into the present by really listening to what they are saying. We don't assume we know what they are telling us just because on the surface their story might be similar to our own, or to that of a previous client we've worked with. We are listening to what they are saying right now, in this moment, using all our senses. And we are not only listening to what they are saying with their voices. We are paying attention to their tone, their silences, their body language, their breathing patterns. It takes very close, attuned listening to understand what a client's bodymind behind their armour is saying, to not be blinded by what the – often very accomplished – armoured version wants us to see. You can learn to do this careful listening for yourself in your yoga practice, and it will eventually follow you off the mat and into all areas of your life, so that when you next feel out of control, you will know how to bring yourself back to a centred place from where to work out what is really going on. Remember that no matter how tumultuous the surface waves, down in its depths the ocean remains calm.

Working in a different medium but from out of a mindset similar to Suzuki's, psychotherapist Wilfred Bion suggested that a therapist should approach every client session 'without memory or desire'.[21] What he meant was that we can only help someone by leaving behind our memory of what we think we know so that we can really learn from what we are being told today. In the same way, we must leave aside our own desire to 'solve' them or to show our own 'cleverness'. Only by stepping away from the desire to effect change can change really happen. Only by the therapist being absolutely in the moment, really listening in to what the client is telling them right here right now, allowing the client to feel their feelings, will that person feel safe enough to change.

Approach your yoga in the same way. Treat your body like a new client – or, if you might find it more helpful, like a small child. Imagine that child facing a new experience, frightened and unsure and holding back, reluctant to embark on something they know nothing about, and which has the potential to cause pain. What would you do? I imagine your instinct would be to gently encourage them to believe that it is going to be all right. You would hold their hand and stay by their side, you would not abandon them.

Why do you deserve less yourself? Bring this attitude to your body, which may similarly be unsure and frightened of pain, muscles clenching. A muscle will never relax if it doesn't feel safe enough to do so. It grips to avoid going too far. So slow things down and really listen to why it is stopping where it is. Promise it you will go at a pace that feels safe – perhaps taking one step forwards, one back. Do the metaphorical equivalent of holding its hand by using a calm and encouraging breath to ease it in deeper. If you show it that you are not going to force it beyond where it feels safe to go, then it will soften. And in softening, it may open a bit more.

Without this attitude an image comes to mind of a mule digging in its heels. No amount of force will cause it to move. If the mule is beaten with a stick, it will just dig in further – remember what we have seen about fear causing us to pull on an inflexible suit of armour as protection against pressure? So ditch the stick, remove the need for armouring, and try a rewarding carrot instead – kindness and understanding as opposed to bullying and punishment. This is how we build trust. This is how we treat children. This is why in psychotherapy we listen, learn and follow as opposed to advise, cajole or lead. See if you can do the same with your yoga.

- **Try a body scan meditation**

In a body scan meditation you lie or sit very still and you allow your mind to wander slowly and gently through different parts of your body, tuning in to each one, resting your awareness in each part – the big toe on your left foot, the next toe, the next, the skin on the top of the foot, the arch of the foot, the heel and so on, up through the entire body, external and internal elements given careful, kind attention, tuning in, noticing how each part is feeling today. Some will be numb, or feel non-existent. Some will feel inseparably fused to other parts. Some will feel tired or aching or itchy. None are judged; each just has a soft light of attention shone upon it, giving it the chance to have its say, to experience feeling like it matters and is not ignored.

You can do a body scan meditation for yourself, or there are many recordings and apps you can download if you would like to listen to someone else guiding you.

This practice establishes trust, develops self-awareness, teaches us to prioritise and notice the intelligence of the body, reminding

Spinning Out of Control

us that it too matters and can make decisions. It also strengthens our interoception – our ability to sense ourselves (see next page). This is important because weak interoception can increase feelings of dissociation – not quite in your own body, not quite in control.

As you work with this practice, you will naturally take its lessons into your more active practices. You will get into the habit of checking in not just with the overall pose, but with each part of your body experiencing the pose in its own way. For Jenny, being able to work through all of her issues by acknowledging them each in turn has given her the confidence to tackle all that life throws at her. This practice can help you in similar ways.

A body scan meditation also strengthens what is known as the 'observer' self (more of this later), the part of you that can step outside of the fray and notice what is going on without getting caught up in momentary sensations.

- **Heighten concentration with a challenging posture**

An alternative way to help yourself notice every little nuanced response is to go to the opposite extreme and really challenge yourself with a very complex posture. For example, standing twists like *parivrtta trikonasana* (revolved triangle) require all parts of the body to both individualise and work seamlessly together, and call on you to move your focus from area to area as you encourage your body into them.

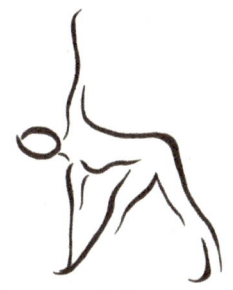

Parvritta Trikonasana

We saw earlier how committing to a regular yoga practice can be an important part of self-care and nurturing. Another benefit of regular practice is that commitment can keep you from spiralling, and make you feel more in control of your own life. This is because for at least a few minutes each day not only do you know where you will be and what you will be doing, but you are also conferring with your body and listening to its messages of support.

A regular practice provides a still point in a turning world, tethering you to something solid amidst the chaos.

Interoception

Interoception is the ability to sense what's going on inside your skin. It's the sensation in the bladder that tells you that you need to go to the loo, the pull of a heavy eyelid that lets you know it's time to sleep; on a slightly more subtle level, it's the fluttering in your tummy indicating that you are excited or the insistent drumming of your heart telling you that you are frightened.

And what about the faint prickle at the back of your neck that advises you not to keep talking to that individual at the bus stop, the slight sinking in your stomach suggesting you might be in the wrong job or relationship? These are very subtle and nuanced messages, but we ignore them to our cost.

We can, though, tune in to them if we give ourselves the time, space and careful attention to do so; and the more we can feel and interpret our physical sensations in this way, the more we get to know ourselves deep down, the more responsive we can be to those messages, allowing us to make better choices to navigate life safely.

Neuroscientific and neurobiological research can now prove to us that our sense of ourselves is anchored in a vital connection with our bodies. Brain scans have revealed that specific areas of the brain, collectively called the pathways of interoceptive awareness,[22] are involved in what's called self-sensing – knowing where we are in space and being aware of the sensations coming from other parts of the body, then connecting these to emotion. The more able we are to detect our interoceptive messages, the better will be our ability to regulate those emotions.

MRIs reveal that people who have suffered trauma have damage in these areas,[23] meaning that if you have suffered trauma you may be particularly likely to feel disconnected from your core being, to feel even less embodied, which can make life feel even more unstable.

Without interoception the body can be a stranger, and a frightening stranger at that. And when emotions are overwhelming and terrifying, the brain blocks them out. But by doing this we also shut down and deaden our capacity to feel a whole range of other emotions, including the 'good' ones.

A yoga practice that trains us to pay careful attention to the most nuanced of internal cues can help us stay in touch with and even reactivate self-sensing areas of the brain.

Neuroscientist Antonio Damasio has described our minds as being located throughout our entire bodies, not just in our brains, and has come to the conclusion that it is only by tuning in to interoception that we can really know what we 'think'.[24] He identified our emotions as being neurally based and the real driving force behind our decision making.[25]

Another neuroscientist Dr Candace Pert is credited with being the person to coin the term 'bodymind'. She too found there to be a biochemical basis for our emotions, describing the body as the 'unconscious mind'.[26]

Dr Stephen Porges, who developed polyvagal theory (see page 80), has called interception our 'sixth sense' and identified it as being crucial to our survival as babies, and to our social behaviour as adults, as it allows us to distinguish safe from dangerous.[27]

Interoception fosters the safe secure base from which we feel able to explore. Agency begins with interoceptive awareness. Without knowing what we feel, we cannot know what we need. And when we don't know what we need, we cannot get our needs met.

So interoception is a prerequisite for safety. You can increase that sense by continually asking yourself to notice what's going on in your body right now. You can get to know what your body likes and doesn't like; in other words, you can befriend it. It can come to feel less like an out-of-control vehicle and more like a safe one.

Yoga Saved My Life
Larisa

Self-harm used to be a harmful meditative practice for me, a very unhealthy way of calming that overwhelming rage rushing through me.

I had rituals around it. Set processes. A discipline. Control. And it was that 'process' and the 'focus' that enabled me to calm my mind, in the most damaging way, and shift my focus.

Spinning Out of Control

Through extending my yoga practice, I began to find new ways to bring that focus, that mindfulness, that release. I discovered new ways of bringing a stillness to the thoughts. New, healthier ways of silencing those demons.

Yoga for me, now, is a holistic experience; it's the mind, the body, the breath and the self. It requires discipline, rituals, processes. And when those overwhelming waves begin to rise within, I know I can take it to my mat, connect to my breath, to my practice and find my way through to still waters again.

And what's more, yoga has given me back an identity. An identity beyond that which I thought I was limited to. It opened up my world and provided me with a community, an extended family. A purpose. It set me on a path.

Yoga has taught me new ways. Better ways. For that I will always be grateful.

Far safer, through an Abbey gallop,
The Stones a'chase—
Than Unarmed, one's a'self encounter—
In lonesome Place—

Ourself behind ourself, concealed—
Should startle most—
Assassin hid in our Apartment
Be Horror's least.

Emily Dickinson
(from 'One need not be a Chamber – to be Haunted')

CHAPTER TWELVE

The Only Way Out Is Through

Yoga Saved My Life
Niché Faulkner

The very first time I felt broken was when I had my miscarriage on my birthday. I blamed myself: if I would have run less or danced less or done all of the shit less and sat my ass down somewhere, my baby would be here and yet there I was staring at that silent screen willing and pleading for God to let me see a heartbeat. I sank into depression.

About a month later, I received an email from a local yoga studio inviting me to participate in a 40-day yoga practice and book study. I could never have imagined that by giving a simple yes, this would be the healing and wholeness I needed in my life. I was broken like, 'Oh shit broken-broken, not eating broken, always crying broken, superrrrrrrr quiet broken.'

The very first day I hit my mat, I didn't know any of the shit the teacher was saying. I remember saying, 'What the phuck' MANY TIMES that day and yet I left with a feeling of understanding allllll of the shit I needed to.

> With a continuous practice, I truly gained a sense of 'It wasn't your fault, Niché'.
>
> Each day after my practice, I learned to ease into my pain, be aware of it, acknowledge my pain and then slowly and surely I eased into letting that shit go.
>
> Hell, yeah #yogasavedmylife and it keeps saving my life every single day.

Do you ever find yourself just doing something on automatic pilot? Always responding to things in the same way? Freud termed this the repetition compulsion;[28] and Einstein apparently said that the definition of madness is doing the same thing over and over and expecting a different outcome. Yet we all do this: go out with the same type of person, find ourselves caught up in the same work dynamic, tell ourselves we definitely will or won't do the same thing again, only to find that the next situation is really just a variation of the last.

In the last chapter we learned about interoception and how checking in with the useful messages our bodies have to impart can give us a more 360-degree view of ourselves, integrating and strengthening our sense of self and bringing a little bit of order to the chaos.

Once we know how to notice our bodies' messages, we can work on responding to them less reactively; on staying with them, not immediately moving on from the ones we don't like and lingering on the ones we do. We need to 'treat those two impostors just the same', to hijack Kipling.

React or Respond

Why do we move away from the feelings or messages we don't like? Daniel Kahneman won a Nobel Prize for his work on the psychology of decision-making.[29] He identified that the avoidance of pain is a far greater motivator than the attraction of pleasure. If you think about it, that makes evolutionary sense; our need to survive and avoid things that threaten our survival are bound to take priority over the pursuit of pleasure, which is a luxury in comparison to the very real need to stay alive. We can see this animal instinct in every creature – from the most basic of amoebic cells upwards, all creatures recoil from pain.

We do not, however, have to be slaves to these primeval instincts. We don't need to just react, to grasp for the good, reject the bad. We have something that can help us counter that instinct – the thinking mind. We can allow some of that top-down processing to help us control the more habitual bottom-up response of recoil. We've spent a lot of time looking at how important it is not to let the intellectual, top-down response blind us to the important embodied, bottom-up messaging, but now it's time to remember that we need both; that the system works best when we balance things out and use all the tools we have at our disposal.

Recent psychotherapeutic theory, informed by neurobiological research,[30] is discovering that it is by connecting to deep emotion, learning to identify, express and manage our emotions, that deep transformation can happen. But that only happens when we feel safe. A good therapist can help create that safety, as can a compassionate, aware yoga practice.

Yoga strengthens both bottom-up and top-down processing AND reinforces the teamwork between them. It teaches us to notice the

The Only Way Out Is Through

feelings and then to pass them through a filter, a neutral observer if you will, to take stock of the message and choose how to respond most usefully. It teaches us how to create a pause, create time to choose what to do next. A real, conscious choice as opposed to an unconscious, habitual reaction.

Psychotherapist, existentialist and concentration-camp survivor Viktor Frankl said: 'Between stimulus and response there is a space. In that space is our power to choose our response. In our response lies our growth and our freedom.'[31]

How do we create and work with this space, or pause?

• Holding poses

Effort and strain like those experienced when you practise yoga manifest in three different spheres – physical pain, emotional upset and negative thinking. Physical and emotional pain are processed through the same neuroanatomical systems, which can make them confusing to decipher. Staying in a pose for longer than you might normally, holding it beyond the point where it feels comfortable, gives you a chance to be with those difficult feelings and to work with them.

You can explore this idea in any pose, but something that you find a little bit challenging will give you more to work with. *Virabhadrasana* 2, for example, is not too complicated yet asks a lot of you physically; the larger muscles of both the legs and the arms are put under strain so to remain there requires both strength and flexibility. By holding, and holding, and holding a bit more, you can observe, examine and be curious about your emotional and mental reactions when you cannot – amoeba-like – just move on and away from the source of the suffering but instead have to bear it beyond the point of comfort.

As you hold you may realise that after a couple of breaths your legs are starting to ache, your arms are getting heavy, your breathing is perhaps becoming more laboured and your mind probably starts getting in on the action, telling you that it is time to move on, away from discomfort, and into the next pose.

You are going to challenge this habitual response, and in challenging it, you may encounter some resistance. This can take many forms but I'm going to guess that your mind takes you deep into one of two stories.

Perhaps, first story, you start hating your teacher, for keeping you there. All the dislike of the pain engendered gets projected outwards to an external cause of blame – the teacher.

Or perhaps you chose a second story. You start hating yourself, telling yourself you are weak, that this is because you don't practise enough, and worry that others will judge you for your lack of fortitude. All your dislike of the pain is internalised, and as it seeks to find blame, you find yourself, to be the most obvious recipient.

Now imagine that there might be a third response. Pause here in the discomfort, and perhaps your body can tell its own story, its own truth of what is, rather than the story you have been forcing it to sign up to all this time.

In time you come to understand that all that is happening is a very natural urge to move away from pain and towards pleasure, and that that urge doesn't, in fact, have to be acted upon; that actually you are able to remain there in the discomfort without having to 'do' anything. This tightrope in the midst of rejection and grasping is the difficult bit. You can balance there by letting it be, by accepting that this moment will pass, that it is temporary. You can use this moment to see what the discomfort can teach you. You have already noticed one tendency – to blame

The Only Way Out Is Through

inwards or outwards. Perhaps there are further lessons that can be learned. Be curious. What is my reaction to this pose trying to teach me? How do I face challenge and change?

Eventually you may notice how those responses which feel so powerful in the moment, very soon mutate and transform into something else. Nothing lasts for ever, everything shape-shifts. Like the flowing and evolving liquids in a lava lamp, feelings emerge from the background, take shape, come to the foreground, loom to the front of the lamp's glass, grow huge and insistent for a moment, then gently break up as you watch them, receding and changing shape and intensity. Use the pause you have created to watch and learn from the shapes and feelings that are now pressing their noses up against the glass of your awareness.

You may be surprised by what you find: some strong sensations, some weak, some numb areas. Which is harder to bear? The silence or whisper of the areas you cannot feel, or the shouting of the areas you feel too much? This is your chance to explore, to focus on those areas, which may signify a defence you didn't know was there. Might those physical blocks be representative of emotional blocks? By connecting to the strong emotions that arise we can update those internal working models we've been ruled by for too long.

By focusing on these areas of physical stuckness and pain, you can see them as the portal into your stuck emotions. Imagine you are sending your breath, full of care and attention, into these areas, unleashing the energy held there, allowing this energy to flow to areas that were previously starved of it, cut off from it by the psycho-physical blocks. When I do this I have a visualisation that comes to me. I get an image of a waterfall unblocking and its waters flooding through to those arid, desert-like parts of my body, finally getting to slake their thirst after years of dryness. The water allows new life to flood to the previously numb or painful areas, while simultaneously releasing the tension that has been held in the parts that have been hanging on tight, keeping the dam in place.

What holding poses can nurture in us is resilience, a bit of a buzz word at the moment. As is tolerance, especially the ability to tolerate change. You may even learn to accept that the only way out of these seeming dead ends is by going through them – as Niché articulates. You cannot bypass the pain without creating other types of pain. Think of the energy it takes to create a dam big enough to hold back a waterfall. Think of the circuitous routes you must take to get round it another way because you are so afraid of going over the top, of being swept away by the force of the water. Think of all the energy you would release and use for better things if you weren't using it to build and hold and bypass an unnecessary dam.

It is in that moment of pause that you face fear. You face yourself. You cannot hide from it any longer. And you might be surprised by what you find. You will almost certainly learn that you are more resilient than you thought, physically and emotionally. Your view of yourself may shift slightly. You may find that off the mat you are more able to accept the present moment, more able to tolerate discomfort in other parts of your life.

As we hold, as we allow the pain, thoughts and emotions to arise, and as we observe our reactions to these, we are developing an 'observing self'. This observing self is a phenomenon fundamentally important both to psychotherapy and to yogic philosophy. It is a quality strengthened by many of the yoga practices, but is most obviously targeted in meditation.

The Only Way Out Is Through

- **Meditate**

Yoga, done mindfully, is a moving meditation. We looked, earlier, at a body scan meditation, in which we paid attention to each body part in turn. Sitting meditation, though, is perhaps the most familiar image that comes to mind when we think of meditation: that image of the serene yogi sitting in lotus position, the pinnacle of calm beatitude.

Just as holding a pose helps you notice – and press pause on – your automatic, unthinking responses, so too in meditation you can practise not getting involved in feelings, stories and reactions, but instead learn to watch them happen. In doing so, you develop a part of you that I like to imagine as the responsible adult not drawn into the playground fighting of the less-conscious selves.

In therapy this idea is known as the observing ego, outlined by the early psychoanalysts of the first half of the twentieth century. In yoga it goes back somewhat further, to at least 2,000 years ago, and to an ancient sage, Patanjali, who described what is known in Sanskrit as *drashtri*, commonly translated as the seer. This seer or 'the one who sees' can watch the mind without falling into the trap of believing or interacting with the thoughts therein.

Many of my clients have told me they have tried meditation but gave up because they weren't any good at it. But none of us is any good at it. That's the point. It is a practice; we keep at it. At the gym, you would start with a weight that you could lift fairly easily for just a couple of times. It would make your arm hurt; but the next time you went you might be able to lift the weight three or four times. Or use a heavier one. In meditation we work the mind as you would work your arm in the gym; we observe the 'noise' of our thoughts and, every time we notice we have been carried away by them, we bring the focus back. As with your arm in the gym, the more repetitions of this 'bringing back' that we do, the more the 'muscle' of observation gets worked, getting stronger over time.

Way back in the anxiety chapter we came across a description of the purpose of yoga: to 'still the fluctuations of the mind'. We can think of these fluctuations as ripples on a lake, or clouds flitting across a blue sky. The seer or observing self is the calm depths of the lake or the unchanging blue sky above those clouds that sees them go past but remains unaffected. In meditation we practise seeing ripples or clouds as they really are – fleeting and transitory. Like physical sensations and emotional responses in our yoga postures.

Psychotherapy and yoga use different language, but their methods and aims are closely related. Both hold up a mirror to our internal worlds. Both are trying to help us reach a state of equanimity. Yoga teaches us not to reject the unpleasant, nor grasp for or cling to the pleasant, but to make room for whatever is there; to resist the impulsive move towards like/dislike and instead to dwell in observer mode.

A psychotherapist will do the same. They will encourage a client to stay with their difficult feelings by, among other things, helping them see their unconscious internal working models play out, observe in which situations they arise and learn not to respond in the same old ways again and again. In yoga and meditation, we can similarly sit, or hold a pose, and watch each feeling, thought and emotion arise – without reacting. This is a powerful tool, stopping us from being governed by unconscious patterns and giving us a choice to respond differently.

The Only Way Out Is Through

Why Cultivate an Observing Self?

On a practical level, MRI scans can now prove scientifically what the yogis have always known – that meditation and the emotional transformations that come alongside it can actually change your brain.[32] Meditation can re-sculpt neural pathways and promote growth in the brain. Crucially, the areas most affected are those that relate to mental health.

Less objectively measurable, but no less important, is what cultivating the pause, and the observer that comes along with it, brings to our daily existence: control. Given that we often don't have as much control as we might like over circumstances in the outside world, the only option we have available is to control our reactions to them. If we feel strong and resilient internally, then we are more likely to look on external challenges as opportunities to grow and change and overcome, rather than be struck down by them.

When I began yoga, when in a pose I found difficult, I would grit my teeth, screw up my face, curse the teacher, myself, yoga and the world, and count the seconds till I could come out of it. I don't think I learned anything beyond just how impatient and full of anger I was. Those were useful things to recognise but greater insight came after a few years of this uncomfortableness. It finally dawned on me that there might be another way to get through it, one that didn't involve my brain just working overtime to project myself forwards to a time when I would no longer have to endure this agony. I started telling myself that I was going to be in the pose for another twenty minutes and I would just have to find a way to be with it, that this current pain was perhaps as good as it got and that in another five minutes it was only going to get worse. I would have to find a way to manage as opposed to fight the pain. Gradually, I began to soften. I yielded into the pose. I would do a body scan, taking my awareness and my breath to each complaining joint and muscle in turn and consciously ask them to let go, to surrender to the experience, to gravity, to allow the floor to take the weight, find what support I could, trust I could stop gripping. It worked. Not instantly – I'm not a saint, I'm a grumpy, impatient human who doesn't like pain – but slowly, gradually I became more used to just being curious about the pain, adjusting my breathing and my expectations and learning to lean into it. Then, when the instruction to move on came not twenty minutes but twenty seconds later, it felt like a bonus, like no time at all had gone past and I saw that not only had I survived it, I'd found the time in it to be really informative and actually not nearly as painful as my brain had been telling me it was. Before long, this ability to yield was making itself apparent in other areas of my life. When I am stuck underground in a packed Tube train, for instance, instead of allowing steam to build behind the ears, I try to find my seat, both literal and metaphorical, to soften into it, tell myself I am here for the duration so I might as well make myself comfortable, and I focus on my breathing. The mechanical jolt, when it does come, of the Tube restarting, therefore brings a corresponding jolt of pleasure that we are moving on so quickly.

What you learn about yourself on the mat or with your therapist does gradually start to seep into life off the mat, outside the therapy room. You develop an ability to stay with discomfort, to apply forensic witnessing of what is really going on inside, to increase your own resilience and tolerance. With greater self-knowledge come greater self-confidence and self-esteem. Old habits, patterns, beliefs are easier to see and therefore easier to challenge with your new-found strength.

The Only Way Out Is Through

Yoga Saved My Life
Andrea Megale Vassileou

In 2000 I began work in an architectural practice in London: my dream job, but the pressure was making its way from the office to home. I thought I was happy, but was always anxious: sleeping less and less, exhausted. I felt I needed more than the prestige and money.

I decided to try yoga and went to an *ashtanga shala*. This practice was like a dance, a strong, graceful and powerful dance. My body, mind and my soul were taken. I was finding my way home. I started to practise twice a week at the *shala* and constantly at home.

I used to bombard my teacher with questions until one day she asked, 'Andrea, why don't you do teacher training?' I looked at her wide-eyed. 'Me?? I am an architect. I have my career.' She replied, 'But are you happy, Andrea?' This question hit me hard!

One day I woke up and it was clear. I wanted to teach yoga. I wanted to be able to make yoga and meditation happen in other people's lives. It was as if everything in my life before brought me to this point of fulfilment and happiness. No more doubts. Everything had finally fallen into place.

Yoga cures what need not be endured and endures what cannot be cured.

B. K. S. Iyengar

CHAPTER THIRTEEN

Take a Leap of Faith

Yoga Saved My Life
Indrayani

I was in hospital after a suffering a complete breakdown. My heart had actually stopped beating and my soul was floating in space saying 'Hi' to God.

I never was rooted or particularly grounded. This Earth. This body. Everything was so strange.

My range of emotions was so big and my senses so wide I felt so much but I couldn't handle it. There was no vessel for all this stuff: my body was a stranger to me, I didn't feel at home in it.

So, from the age of thirteen I started to use drugs and alcohol; battled with bulimia nervosa, anorexia and extreme sports to FEEL ME.

But the body is no unbreakable machine and it eventually broke down when I was twenty. I knew: if I wanted to live I had to change.

I went to a yoga ashram far away from society. In *savasana* I had the same feeling I had in hospital. God was there. But God was in me. And I felt that within my body. Within my powerful beating heart. Within every breath. In my skin. In my veins. I felt ME.

> I cried. And laughed. I felt.
>
> Now, I do not need drugs or extremes that damage me to feel me any more. I turned a corner, living clean and healthy, allowing me to give birth to my little boy six years ago.
>
> Yoga is my key. My anchor to this fantastic world and body. Grounded. I found my home.
>
> And for sure sometimes it's hard here on Earth but I love it. I nourish my body, to allow me to enjoy this life… this life is a big WOOOOW and I am so thankful that I realised that. And I have yoga to thank for that.

I'm going to take my own pause here (see what I did there?) to stop and reflect a moment on what we have learned so far. We've seen how yoga can help us manipulate our nervous systems and along with them the myriad other internal workings of the bodymind. We've seen how integrated all these systems are, how minor changes in one part can lead to major changes in another. We've harnessed our yoga to rouse us from depression, calm us from anxiety and stress, give us courage when we feel like a victim, and translate unhelpful outer defences into inner strength and resilience. And we've started looking at creating mindful pauses in which to explore our attitudes to pain in the service of starting to rewire our most innate and ingrained physical, neural, emotional and unconscious habits and ways of working.

Are you sold? Have I made a good case? I hope so, but do you know what? It doesn't really matter if not. Because one of the many amazing things about yoga is that it will work whether you believe any of this 'stuff' or not. It will work its magic even if you actively reject it all and just want a good workout, or a space for calm relaxation. You don't need to know or believe a word.

Yoga will be quietly going about its work anyway, as it has for millennia. I started out telling you what an ancient practice this is, how the early practitioners had nothing but their own self-study and experience to draw on, yet they knew it worked. And now modern science is able to prove their findings more measurably.

This scientific backup may be validating and reassuring to some, yoga's ancient roots may be what sways others and some may just be happy to have found something that 'works' for them and don't wish to delve any deeper. These are all understandable positions.

However, I feel pulled to talk about something that maybe transcends whichever depth of engagement you bring to your practice. It's a hard one to put into words – and in itself that seems to be an argument for including it; so much of what is important in life does not reside in the world of words or rationality but instead inhabits the realm of intuitive knowing, of feeling, of instinct. And it is in that realm – non-verbal, spiritual, ineffable, whatever term you want to use – that yoga can be particularly powerful; that area where words or logic elude us but somehow the yoga speaks for us.

I've talked a lot about the symbolism of the postures, of how they help us – without the need for words – to embody, inhabit, give expression to, and become other selves: our inner warrior, our inner mountain, our inner child and so on.

The posture that, for me, represents this slightly more esoteric chapter is one that epitomises the un-pin-down-able nature of all of this. *Hanumanasana* (scissor splits) symbolises taking a leap of faith into the unknown; into trust; into believing that yoga will catch you, be your safety net, show you that it will all be all right.

There is also an element of letting go, surrendering into the pose, into what is available to you here and now, allowing yourself to believe 'you got this'. A classic epic text of India, the *Bhagavad Gita*,[33] exhorts us to do what we can and leave the rest to God. You can replace 'God', of course, with any word and concept that resonates with you – fate, the universe, nature, flow, a higher power, truth, light, consciousness, your better self; the essence of what it conveys is that we must recognise what we can and can't do and also that – ironically – we are likely to go further if we can give up our attachment to the outcome and enjoy the journey.

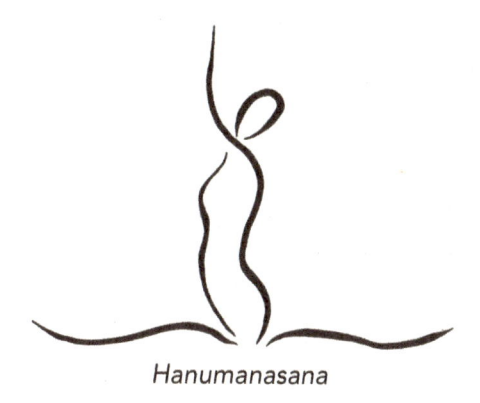

Hanumanasana

Hanuman's Leaps

Hanuman, the monkey, is a hugely important figure in Hindu mythology. He is the child of the wind and a mortal, which makes him a wonderful bridge between the spirit and the material world.

He symbolises the bridging of two worlds – the unifying force underpinning all yoga – his role in another epic story, the *Ramayana*, in which he first takes one enormous and risky leap across the ocean from India to Sri Lanka to rescue King Rama's beloved Queen Sita after she has been kidnapped. In another story, he leaps from southern India to the Himalayas to fetch a herb that will save the life of King Rama's brother, Lakshman.

Symbolically, this tells us that with enough devotion and faith in your heart you can overcome seemingly impossible obstacles in the service of someone you love; that having the courage to leap into the unknown can unite lovers and even confront death.

The pose itself resembles a leap – this is the splits, remember – so requires a lot of the body in terms of strength and flexibility, and asks for bravery in the face of perhaps feeling like you are literally being split apart. The journey towards the full expression of this pose may be a long one; many of us have to accept that we will never reach its final destination. The learning comes from that acceptance. And from going for it anyway.

It's a journey that can bring great insight, requiring as it does huge amounts of patience, kindness and good old legwork (pun intended). Here's what's needed:

- Length in your hamstrings.
- Opening in your hips.
- Core strength to keep your torso upright.
- Humility to accept the support of props.
- Mindfulness and care: you may find you can lower further into the pose if you externally rotate your hip, but what if that causes your pelvis to move out of its safe position?
- Honesty: is your need to 'get there' greater than the need for safer, slower progress? If so, what does that tell you about you and your need to cheat, or your perfectionism, or the value you place on achieving the appearance of the pose over proper alignment?
- Acceptance to learn that it is not about getting the posture 'right' – it's about focusing on developing a healthier relationship with your body; can you remember the lessons of *ahimsa* and self-care and compassion?

Take a Leap of Faith

In *Hanumanasana* you are leaping over your old boundaries and finding new lands of possibility. The physical expansiveness of the pose represents the expansiveness you can feel if you have faith; faith in yourself or in a higher power. It is not just Hanuman's own story that carries a valuable message, but the story of the pose itself and how it manifests in your bodymind. It's about faith but it's also about reaching for what may seem impossible and gaining the self-belief that you will get there – or that you will be okay if you don't.

As we have seen, yoga in the modern West can sometimes seem to be only concerned with how it can make you feel physically and emotionally in the here and now of this bodymind and this material world. This is not at all the full picture, and if you would like to learn more, you may want to engage with the philosophical and historical texts that debate what yoga is, has been, and can be, and to whom. The *Bhagavad Gita*, mentioned earlier, is a good place to start, and there are many other symbolically rich texts to discover.

Whether through the written word or the physical practice of postures, breathing and meditation, many people, including some of those whose stories we see here, find yoga to be a conduit into a more spiritual or meaningful place. We can all connect to our own spirituality through better connection with ourselves. Perhaps yoga might be your medium for doing so.

Yoga Saved My Life
Joseph Armstrong

I was a drug dealer. I lied a lot. I hurt myself and others. I cheated. I stole. I was existentially morbid and inconsolable.

Yoga Saved My Life

I could not make peace with my place in the world.

The first time I drank, I got drunk. That was in high school and later, it got serious: weed, ecstasy, coke, and eventually shooting up meth.

Oddly, as I experimented with drugs, I also experimented with yoga. A friend took me to my first class in 2008.

My addictive personality applied to my practice. Though my life was completely unmanageable, I kept showing up to classes. Eventually, my yoga addiction replaced my drug addiction.

I spent so long running from things. There was always some new self-imposed heartbreak. So many years spent hunting what would make me feel good. That chase eventually landed me on death's door. That dark place made me see yoga as a tool to help me restructure my life.

Where once there was doubt, fear and a need for answers, now there is comfort with uncertainty. There is an adventurer's heart. There is a love for possibilities and the questions that creation poses.

In recovery lingo, we say: if you wanna keep what you have, you have to give it away. That's why I've devoted myself to sharing yoga. I was a destructive force in the world for so long, but something miraculous occurred when I surrendered to powers greater than myself. I can help others now. This is my sacred responsibility.

And if the body does not do fully as much as the soul?
And if the body were not the soul, what is the soul?
Walt Whitman

CHAPTER FOURTEEN

I'm Angry

Yoga Saved My Life
Danny D. Holmes

My journey of yoga started in a place called jail.

I ended up in Walton HMP Liverpool on charges of Section 20 and affray – basically gang violence.

In jail I took yoga and mindfulness classes and read all the books from the library I could get my hands on. When speaking with the monk who ran the classes he said to me he saw one of two visions for me: either gang leader or spiritual teacher…

After quitting gang life on release I took four yoga classes a week plus self-practice, got a job teaching yoga around the world and have plans to set up a yoga studio in the Mediterranean.

So yes, yoga saves lives and gives eternal positivity and spiritual awareness. I love my life and I love the universe for giving me this opportunity.

Like they say… The universe delivers when the person is ready. *Om namah shivaya.*

Woody Allen apparently once said that he never gets angry, he grows a tumour instead. This, like Allen himself, can be a contentious issue, especially when phrased quite so simplistically. Yet it speaks to a truth that many of us don't really want to confront: that our bodies can represent our emotions, even to the point of physical illness, just as Indrayani told us in the last chapter.

When we cannot verbally express our truths, sometimes our bodies do it for us. We've already looked at the close interaction between the nervous system and our emotions, so it should come as no surprise that such a powerful emotion as anger is going to both originate from a very deep place <u>and</u> have powerful expressions and consequences.

We've seen how our defences – whether represented physically or mentally – work as a protection against feeling, and we employ these in many different ways. We can go for the repression option, where we refuse to acknowledge any anger and lock it away inside; there it can eat away as resentment or leak out as passive aggression or martyrdom. Or we can go to the opposite extreme and act out with unmediated fury, even violence. Neither is helpful. Repression has been shown to increase physiological – and also therefore emotional – stress with all its negative consequences, while unbridled raging has been shown to lead to high blood pressure and heart attack[34] – and of course also harms whoever is on the receiving end.

Sometimes we veer wildly between these two responses, which only exhausts and confuses us and our physiology (and anyone else involved) even further.

But we don't have to get stuck in one or other of these extremes. Both yoga and therapy can help us find a way back to the centre of the court, where we can learn a less extreme, more healthy way

I'm Angry

of responding to anger. In fact, experiencing and expressing our anger – genuinely and with emotional intelligence – has been scientifically shown to reduce physiological stress and promote healing.[35]

Self-Regulation

Self-regulation provides the lever to control the swing of the pendulum, creating a more manageable swing and stopping it before it gathers so much force and energy that we are rendered powerless. It can stop us from lashing out in irrepressible anger or swinging the other way into denial or physical illness as in the case of Woody Allen's tumour. Managing your emotions more effectively means you cope better with almost any situation life throws at you.

In an ideal world we learn self-regulation as infants through what is initially done via co-regulation. Our caregiver acts as a container for our most unbearable emotions, digests them and feeds them back to us in a more bearable form. It's almost as though we sub-contract out our inability to cope with overwhelming feelings we are not equipped to handle, getting an adult to do it for us. And eventually, through that trusting relationship we master the tools to do it for ourselves. But for so many of us, that doesn't happen, for myriad reasons. Yet a good therapeutic relationship can work in a reparative way by mirroring what a good early relationship should offer.

Yoga too gives us powerful tools for self-regulation. We've seen how it gives us the self-awareness to spot powerful feelings rising, and teaches us to pause and be with those feelings without reacting. Yet another very important tool it provides is awareness and manipulation of the breath, which is a crucial conduit towards mastering self-regulation. An asana practice gently encourages us to deepen our breath – we naturally breathe in more deeply as we challenge ourselves, as we move more actively and as we backbend; while the forward bends, static postures and compassionate resting poses encourage longer, deeper exhalations to balance the changes in the inhale. This happens even if we are not aware of it. But we can make this a far more conscious process, both while moving through the asanas and by including specific breathing exercises in our practice.

Breathing and *Pranayama*

We are probably all familiar with the idea, often learned in childhood, that we can calm our anger by taking ten deep breaths. It may seem simplistic, but clichés often become clichés because they contain a grain of truth. It is interesting how entrenched in us, even in the West, is this knowledge that we can use the breath to moderate our anger.

The breath acts as a mirror, showing the state of our nervous system – we naturally breathe far more shallowly and quickly when stressed, for instance, more deeply when calm; and we can harness it to affect our nervous systems to our benefit.

Prana is the Sanskrit word for our life force or energy, and *pranayama* refers to how we access and harness this energy. The word has come to be used as a somewhat catch-all term for breathing exercises, the breath being the best conduit of *prana* that we have. For simplicity's sake I am using the words interchangeably.

There are many, many *pranayama* practices and, just as with the asanas and how we practise and sequence them, they can be put to specific use and target particular desired effects.

Because the breath and the state of the nervous system are so closely linked, focusing on and manipulating your breathing can

I'm Angry

be powerful, triggering even, so if you are new to yoga it's particularly important to begin gently and mindfully. Ask your teacher to start you off with some awareness exercises and get used to how those make you feel before moving on to anything more complicated, like those below. The following actually manipulate the breath, and are worth considering if anger is an issue.

- **Viloma pranayama**

This is a relatively simple practice and helps you to improve your control of your breath by working with interrupting it.

Viloma means 'against the natural course'. The *viloma* – or interruption – can be practised on either the inhalation or the exhalation or both. It is cooling, regulates energy and helps reduce anxiety. Practising *viloma* on the exhalation is a good regulatory tool to calm anger.

- Start by taking a deep inhalation followed by an exhalation.
- Imagine your lungs are divided into three distinct sections, bottom to top.
- On your next inhalation, breathe in only a third of the way. Imagine your breath filling the lower third of the lungs.
- Pause and hold the breath.
- Now take in another third of the breath, imagining that you are filling the central portion of your lungs.
- Pause and hold again (remember, this is one interrupted breath, not three separate breaths).
- Now allow the final third of the breath to enter, taking it into the top portion of the lungs. Fill yourself right up to the collarbones.
- Pause again at the top of this breath, feeling its fullness, then allow yourself a long, deep, uninterrupted exhalation.

- Repeat a few rounds of this then go back to breathing normally and see how it has left you feeling.

- **Simha mudra pranayama**

In Sanskrit, *simha* means lion and *mudra* means a hand gesture.

- Make your hands into fists, close your eyes, inhale.
- Exhale forcefully from the back of the throat and out through the mouth as though roaring like a lion.
- As you breathe out, stick the tongue out at the same time as taking the eyes skywards, and open the hands and stretch the fingers.
- This releases tension in the hands, jaw, face and neck, all areas that tend to tense up when we are angry. It is a way of letting go – of other people's opinions and of negativity – and it is calming and good for stress reduction.
- It also helps 'give voice' to one's feelings and resentments.
- All of this helps dissipate anger safely and on a physiological level.

- **Sarvangasana**

When it comes to postures that are particularly useful for self-regulation, I would suggest *sarvangasana*. Also known as shoulder stand, it is often referred to as the queen or the mother of postures, such is its efficacy. Iyengar said of it, 'As a mother strives for harmony and happiness in the home, this asana strives for harmony and happiness in the human system.'[36]

Sarva in Sanskrit means 'entire' while *anga* means 'organ' or 'body part'. In other words, this is a pose that has benefits for the entire body. This, alongside it being one of the few postures that can be used either to rouse or to calm the nervous system, makes it a fantastic way to improve self-regulatory skills. Having

I'm Angry

the heels above the heart calms the nervous system, while having the heart above the head improves blood flow, which is energising. Being inverted also reinvigorates the lymph system – which can otherwise become sluggish – helping it to more effectively transport waste products towards the lymph nodes where they can be dealt with. Symbolically, letting go of 'waste' is a good way to think about dealing with anger.

We've talked throughout this book about the idea of being controlled and overpowered by our feelings, and how we might instead try observing as opposed to reacting to them. One way to access this verbally in therapy is to try to reframe the language used. If you say, 'I am angry' it is almost as though you are defining yourself, telling yourself that that is all you are. Try saying, 'I feel angry' instead – that way you can see the separation. Anger, or any emotion, is something temporary that you – the observer – notice yourself feeling but you don't have to be defined or flooded by it. You are not at its mercy, rendered powerless by it, you are merely aware that it is there and that it needs to be acknowledged and worked with.

When we are poised between over- and under-reactivity, we can approach our anger – any emotion, in fact – with curiosity as opposed to judgement. We neither have to ignore it out of fear nor act out in order to get rid of it. If we are not overwhelmed but can retain some ability to observe, then we are more likely to see another's point of view not as attacking, but as having some merit, something that can be absorbed and chewed over without toxicity. The more our 'observer self' comes to understand our own impulses, the more it can then help us to understand others. We may stop seeing their actions only through the prism of our own feelings, and understand instead that they too are motivated by many complex and intertwined forces, which can become less unwieldy if attended to kindly and with understanding. This is *ahimsa*, compassion, at work again.

> ### Yoga Saved My Life
> #### Christine Elaine
>
> I was the quintessential late thirties SuperMum. Corporate America vice-president, two young daughters… and trying to protect those two young daughters from a manic-depressive alcoholic husband.
>
> 'My body protested – I developed multiple allergies, bouts of anxiety and depression; chronic acid reflux, delayed gastric emptying, IBS, insomnia, diffuse muscle spasms and all-over pain. I kept going, ignoring the body's wisdom, began taking prescription medication, pain meds, opiate pain meds, Band-Aids over gaping wounds.
>
> Botched trigger-point injections (aimed at relieving the muscle spasms) finally landed me in hospital for five days, with double lung puncture.
>
> 'Death has to be better than this,' I thought.
>
> Two weeks later I signed up for yoga teacher training.
>
> I never intended to teach. Fifth class in, something SHIFTED. My thoughts changed to 'How can I NOT teach???!!' I completed training, quit my job and worked through an acrimonious divorce.
>
> To feed my soul, I went to India, took and then taught ecstatic dance programmes and Thai yoga massage, learned shamanism and reiki. I taught yoga at YMCAs and high schools and began teaching teachers too.

I'm Angry

At forty-eight, I began saying 'Yes' to the opportunities the universe presents.

Yoga didn't just change my life, it totally TRANSFORMED it and actually GAVE me a LIFE to live, vs an existence.

To an ever freer and joyous new Phoenix from THOSE ashes! Stay well. Stay strong. Stay positive. Stay Present.

The test of a first-rate intelligence is the ability to hold two opposed ideas in the mind at the same time, and still retain the ability to function.

F. Scott Fitzgerald

CHAPTER FIFTEEN

I Don't Like Conflict

YoYoga Saved My Life
Robyn Childers

I woke up from a coma fifteen years ago today. I'd been lying in ICU for four days on a ventilator after an intentional drug overdose. The pain I'd been desperately trying to escape seemed more powerful than ever.

For the first year that followed this incident, most of my thoughts and feelings weren't positive. Not even close. I was just trying to survive myself long enough to come into some deeper healing, and most days, wasn't even sure I really wanted to make it.

No matter how hard it got, though, there was one persistent thought that kept me hanging in there: maybe I was here to do something.

Despite my greatest attempts to die, somehow I survived this horrific experience. Doctors said they had no medical explanation for why.

So, what if, just maybe, there was something more for me to do here?

I found yoga and began to develop a practice.

Through yoga, I'm no longer a prisoner to my doubts, fears, cravings and aversions. As I stood in sacred space

I Don't Like Conflict

> this morning, remembering my awakening from death's grip, I've never felt more grateful to be here, alive and free.
>
> If you have not left this world yet, then there is more for you to do. Make amends, forgive yourself, learn from your mistakes. And then begin again.

One of the reasons that some of us have a problem with anger is because we don't like conflict – we don't want to rock the boat. We tend to see anger and conflict as synonymous. Yet conflict can be the spark that ignites an idea, the crucible of creativity. The truth is that the absence of conflict is often not harmony, but apathy. It is a withdrawing from the creativity and blossoming that can result from integrating different viewpoints. But if we can see both those viewpoints as valid and if we can draw from them, as opposed to shutting them down out of fear, then they can become doorways to new, more expansive ways of being, of approaching life differently. Yoga can help us find, learn to be comfortable with and draw on that creative tension.

We've already seen how yoga helps us self-regulate, enabling us to spend more time in the vast middle ground that lies between extremes. But oh, how most people wince at the thought of being neutral, seeing nothing but blandness there!

Nothing could be further from the truth. Perhaps it helps not to see the middle ground as bland but instead as an exciting third way: the energetic centre from which creativity can pour forth. Let's find a different lens through which to see it.

Picture things not so much as a choice between two, a straight line between two extremes, but as a three-way conversation, like the points of a triangle, or a tripod. A tripod is stable in a way that a single line is not. A tripod, with its central point of stability, in many ways represents the balance we are searching for. Or think of a pyramid and how it represents power and integration.

- **Explore trikonasana**

Trikonasana – triangle posture – beautifully embodies this notion of creative tension. It moves us beyond the restrictions of polarity, to the very edge of our abilities, drawing on the possibility and potential of both sky and Earth, while simultaneously making us ever more conscious of our inner core, firing up creativity.

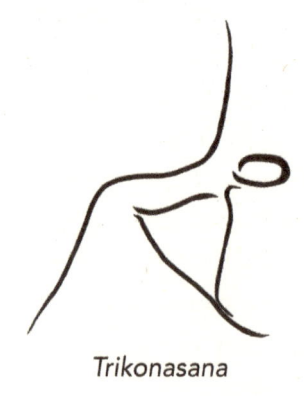

Trikonasana

There are three main triangles contained within this pose:

- The triangle connecting us to the Earth via our legs, with the ground as one side of the triangle and the two feet marking the beginning and end of the side of the triangle. The legs themselves make up the two other sides, with the pelvic floor as the third point.
- The triangle with the pelvic floor as one point and the two hands, one reaching to the sky, one reaching to the Earth, as

the others, connected via the outstretched arms whose midpoint is the chest.
- The triangle with the spreadeagled hands as two of the angles, with imaginary sides connecting them to the third angle at the crown of the head, itself reaching beyond and out into the ether.

Symbolically, we can see the lower triangle as representing a solid foundation consisting of the Earth and our legs; the triangle formed by the chest and arms as representing a connection to the inner self; and at the head a less corporeally grounded, largely ethereal and more spiritually minded one. We can see this as echoing our evolving consciousness and development from the material to the immaterial, earthly to spiritual; and in terms of productive conflict and useful conversation, different perspectives and different forms of awareness.

Within this pose there is always an experience of extending outwards to the world and to your potential via the reaching motion of the fingertips, crown and feet, and yet there is always a connection to a third point that creates connection between the opposites while drawing you inwards and anchoring you. You are creating a pressure, but a useful, productive pressure, from both outside and in, resulting in a posture symbolising stability, grace and potential.

Physiologically, too, *trikonasana* works us hard:

- It strengthens and lengthens the muscles of the waist, abdominals, hamstrings, quads, knees and ankles.
- It opens and creates space and flexibility in the spine and the hips.
- You need to engage the core, draw energy inwards, even while your extremities are reaching outwards.

- Your feet are pushing down into the earth while also pushing away from each other, as though to increase the distance between them, all while your inner thighs are drawing upwards.
- Your arms are reaching away from each other in opposite directions, one skywards, one ground wards, meaning the shoulder girdle has to strongly engage its muscles, drawing the shoulder blades in towards each other for mutual support, as well as downwards.

- **Find other triangles**

You can see that there is a lot going on in *trikonasana*. There's barely a part of the body, inside and out, that isn't engaged. And the breath and the *drishti* (gaze point) are too. The mind also has to remain focused if you are not to topple over.

You need all of these qualities in almost all postures. Play with some others and find the triangles, the creative tension, within. Below are some to get you thinking – but you can, of course, use some of that creativity and curiosity that your *trikonasana* has engendered and find your own triangles within less obvious poses.

- *Ardha chandrasana* (half-moon) – taking *trikonasana* on to one leg to add complexity with the element of balance.

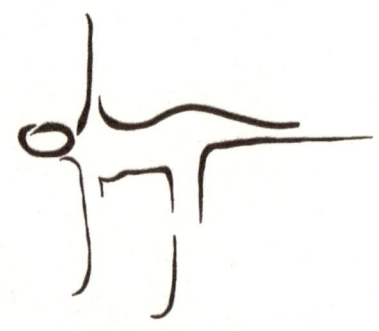

Ardha Chandrasana

I Don't Like Conflict

- *Parsvottanasana* (intense side stretch)– taking it into a different orientation and adding complexity with a less stable hip position.

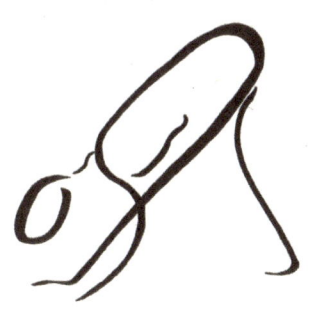

Parsvottanasana

- *Ardha vasisthasana* (half side plank)– challenging your equanimity by adding a need for extra strength.

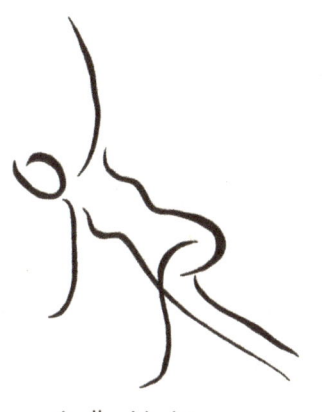

Ardha Vasistasana

- *Parsvakonasana* (extended side angle) – seeing what asymmetry adds to the pose by having the two legs doing different things.

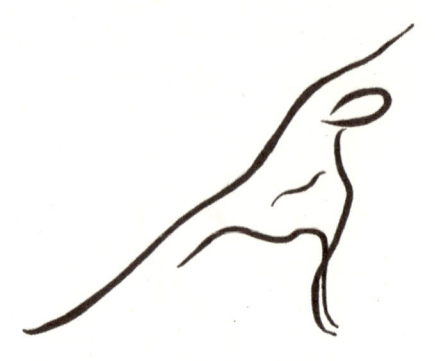

Parsvakanasana

- *Padmasana* (lotus) – making yourself more stable by seeing what having a different 'floor' – your sitting bones – brings to your concentration levels.

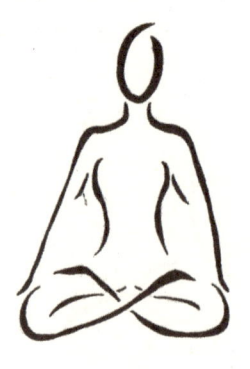

Padmasana

- **Strengthen your core**

Many yoga postures will help you strengthen your core, but some are particularly good for it. Experiment for yourself as to which best enable you to access this area. You may want to look at *vasisthasana* (plank), *navasana* (boat) or *pinca mayurasana* (elbow stand).

I Don't Like Conflict

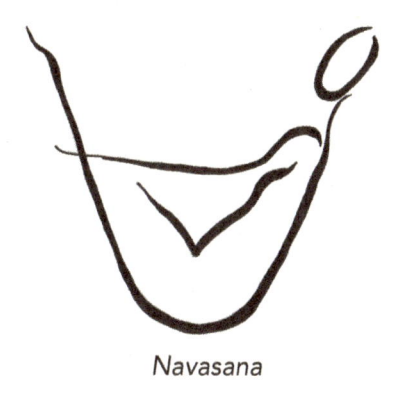

Navasana

- **Expand your *pranayama* practice**

You may have noticed that as we've got further into the book there is slightly less about asana and slightly more about meditation and breathing. This echoes a yoga practice itself which will generally move from the grosser – more physical – to the more subtle over the course of the session, moving the larger limbs quite actively at first, refining it down to a more precise focus on small physical elements towards the end, before moving on to breathing exercises and finishing with meditation.

As you get more and more familiar with deeper layers of yourself through yoga, or as you perhaps become more and more curious about the deeper levels of yoga itself, you may find yourself spending more time exploring the myriad *pranayama* practices.

Triangles and groups of threes underpin so many concepts, both concrete and abstract – on page 173 there is more on about how often they pop up in different arenas including yogic, spiritual and psychotherapeutic. They seem to foster creativity and wholeness, their balancing symbolism offering a nuance that can be all-encompassing as opposed to excluding.

Discovering and exploring a third way is a path out of seeing conflict as only ever being negative; a way of incorporating and integrating our own inner contradictions and thereby finding a more collaborative way of working through the difficulties we may have with others. This could help some of the anger we looked at in the last chapter to be experienced and expressed through creative means rather than aggression or repression.

I am writing this at a very polarised time where there is a tendency for different factions – Brexiteers and Remainers, climate-change activists and deniers, Covid anti- and pro-vaxxers – to be very firmly entrenched in their own camps. Kleinian splitting externalised and writ large. I think we can all see how destructive that is. If we could try viewing things through another's lens, listening compassionately to opposing viewpoints, then we may all start to edge towards the middle of the court and find that third angle from which to explore our differences empathically and constructively.

Yoga Saved My Life
Shannon Kaneshige

I have been practising on and off since I was six years old, but never really felt like I could call myself a yoga practitioner because I didn't feel like there was space for me. I didn't look like the people on the yoga DVDs and on YouTube and my body didn't look like theirs when I went into asana. I thought it meant I wasn't doing it right.

I'd walk into a studio in an attempt to learn the 'right way' and get the look, the you-don't-belong-here look, and I'd turn around and walk right back out.

Once I met a fat yoga instructor and found a community of fat practitioners it was so incredibly freeing. I learned that I had the ability to make asana fit me. I found the deep beauty of a personal practice that went beyond asana.

I trained as a teacher so I could offer representation for my fellow fat practitioners and my fellow non-binary practitioners. Now I work to help others learn to take up space both on and off the mat.

Yoga is my safe place. A space where I can reconnect with my body after years of fighting it and being told it is wrong.

Yoga has helped me find moments of patience and calm as I learn to parent a cancer survivor. By no means has it been a magic cure-all, but it has taught me to sit with discomfort and even find moments of peace in it.

Three Is a Magic Number

In psychotherapy:
- Id, ego, superego
- Victim, persecutor, rescuer
- Adult, child, parent
- Dependency, independence, interaction
- Oedipal triangle

In yoga:
- *Tamas, raja, satva*
- *Vata, pitta, kapha*
- *Ida, pingala, sushumna*

- Strength, balance, flexibility
- Mind, body, spirit
- Mind, body, breath

In religion:
- Father, Son, Holy Ghost
- Brahma, Vishnu, Shiva
- The Three Kings
- Three-headed gods and goddesses
- Three Inca deities – sun, moon, storm

Three represents strength in Taoism, loyalty and respect in China, while in Egypt a pyramid's base represents the body, the sides represent spiritual attempts and the apex symbolises the union between human and God.

Yoga Saved My Life
Lindsey McCracken

I found yoga during recovery from an eating disorder and exercise addiction that has plagued me for most of my life.

For the first time in my life, I have found a space to connect my mind, body and spirit. While I am on my yoga mat, nothing but peace is present – a welcome break from the mental demons I battle daily.

I Don't Like Conflict

A while back, a wise yogi goddess taught me that my yoga mat is a mirror to my life. I'm not gonna lie, that sounded a bit crazy to me at first. But the longer I'm on this journey called life, and in the yoga practice that God gifted me with, the more I see that to be true.

Finding my voice has allowed me to speak my truth.

I'll be the first to admit, I can be stubborn and defiant. But I also love the people and things in my life with my whole heart. I am sensitive and caring. I don't do anything less than 100 per cent. I am a fighter, a survivor, a warrior, an advocate and fiercely loyal. So much of my life has been spent trying to find my voice, and I will not silence it just to make others comfortable. I require no validation, no approval, no recognition. I am a strong woman and I am proud God made me this way.

Yoga helps me to keep fighting for freedom and truth, even during my darkest times. My practice saved my life, and continues to do so.

Our body and mind are not two, and not one.
If you think your body and mind are two, that is wrong.
If you think that your body and mind are one, that is also wrong.
Our body and mind are both two and one.
Shunryū Suzuki[37]

CHAPTER SIXTEEN

Old Habits Die Hard

Yoga Saved My Life
Terri-Ann Carty

In 2012 I took my life back and quit drinking and drugging.

I had been ravaged by my addictions for over ten years and one morning, after a series of devastating events, I looked in the mirror, not recognising my face, and decided right then and there that I was done. I got to rehab, did all the things that were suggested, but felt like I needed more.

Yoga had been in and out of my life since my twenties and I loved it but my addictions were stronger. After three months of sobriety, I gave myself a gift – I took myself on a yoga retreat. To say that week changed my life would be a major understatement. I knew after that week was over that yoga was in my life to heal me.

Three years after getting sober, I nose-dived into teaching. Today, I spend my days giving back what I have learned. The yoga community has alcoholics too (shocking, I know) and now I sponsor teachers and students. I am beyond grateful for my practice, my sobriety, for living one breath, one day at a time.

Old Habits Die Hard

When you feel a bit low, or a bit chaotic, or stressed, or like you can't cope, what do you normally do? Obviously I'm expecting the answer, 'I do my yoga practice', but I'm guessing, if we're being honest, most of us turn to rather more established habits instead – be that alcohol, smoking, chocolate, coffee, retail therapy, Netflix, social media likes or even a heavy workout session in the gym. Those things can have their place, of course they can, and I'm not saying you won't carry on enjoying those things as well. However, in this chapter I'm going to look at how we might use yoga to think about breaking old habits. Not because we won't want to do those things sometimes – we will – but because it might be nice to have the choice.

A habit tends to be a habit because we just fall into doing it automatically. We don't even think about whether it is really what we need right now, or whether it's a helpful or healthy response; we just do it without our rational brain ever having got involved. It's knee-jerk, automatic pilot – I feel bad, therefore I will do this thing that has always made me feel good in the past. Yoga may eventually come to be one of the things that you turn to instead; but this chapter is not even about pushing that as an option. It's more about using yoga to help you work even more usefully with the small pause that we have discovered can exist in between the feeling and the knee-jerk doing.

Create the pause, learn to tolerate it and we strengthen the observer self who can emerge during that moment. We can now *choose* a response consciously rather than *reacting* unconsciously. Otherwise our habits can become addictions, and eventually the thing we do to make ourselves feel better will instead become something that usurps our power.

Demons

Terri-Ann speaks for so many when she tells of how powerless she felt about her drink and alcohol addictions. We probably all know what it feels like to be pulled towards our own demons, be they sugar, gambling, workaholism, shopping or any of the other props we use to help us manage or suppress strong emotions. When these start to become major players in our lives – when we start to feel that they are controlling us rather than we them – then we need to take action. And that is hard.

The traditional view of addiction being a failure of moral resilience and lack of willpower has – mercifully – been debunked by research showing that it is born of pain and trauma (and we'll look more closely at trauma in the next chapter) and is, in fact, a physiologically understandable attempt to ease that pain.[38]

The path to managing our emotions and pain in a healthier way can be a long and lonely one. It's a path that has very little to do with willpower but a lot to do with everything we've been learning about so far: self-compassion, finding support and understanding from others, improving our ability to self-regulate.

Most of us struggle with that 'pause' we've identified and are learning to elongate. We want to turn to our comforts, because the pause is uncomfortable and gives rise to feelings we'd rather not feel. For some of us, however, that pause is more than just uncomfortable. It's unbearable. People suffering from trauma, for example, have a smaller window of tolerance,[39] so the things that might seem easily bearable to some people are experienced by trauma sufferers at much higher magnitude.

Yoga and Addiction

Addictions are driven by unmet emotional needs. And those needs become mapped within our neural pathways and embedded within our brain chemistry.[40] Our experiences wire our brain circuits, priming them for addiction. Luckily, brain plasticity (adaptability) means that we can rewire them, but it takes work. Work that yoga can help with.

A study trialling yoga for substance-abuse treatment[41] demonstrated that yoga might be able to change brain chemistry. The study found that yoga led to increased levels of GABA in the brain. GABA is a neurotransmitter, and low levels of it are often seen in people with anxiety and depression – conditions that often go alongside addiction.

All the elements of yoga that we've looked at so far have taught you that you can tolerate discomfort and that you have the inner resources and strength to withstand uncomfortable feelings that, in this context, might otherwise make you resort to artificial substances. A good yoga practice can support you to tackle addiction as it incorporates all the lessons we've been learning along the way and the good effects yoga offers: it balances both halves of the nervous system to help self-regulation; works to extend the pause, which allows for both top-down and bottom-up processing to help prevent a knee-jerk reach for the addictive behaviour; and, especially if you have been feeling disempowered by your habit or addiction, enables you to feel more empowered and in control.

The observer self becomes stronger with time and practice and allows you to recognise that whatever feelings arise are transitory and can be borne. And training yourself to be acutely aware of all the physical sensations in different parts of the body can help keep the mind focused on the present moment. This all helps you to let go of the old stories about yourself – I'm useless, I can't manage without my drugs, my chocolate, my work – and makes way for new ones: I can do this; the drugs, my job, my food intake don't define me, my feelings of overwhelm don't define me; all are fleeting, all pass, and I can tolerate them.

Addiction is a coping mechanism. As we find better coping mechanisms through yoga, we have less need of the addiction. As we gain inner strength through our practice, we also gain the strength to confront our habits off the mat.

When you start to make friends with your body, as yoga encourages and enables, when you have learned to listen to it and take it into account, when you have stopped either being frightened of it or bullying it into doing things that may not be helpful, then you can use it as a resource to help you make better choices. To stop the automatic reach for the drink or the food or the drugs.

Neuroscience tells us that the more we do something, the more the neural pathways in our brain come to expect us to keep doing that thing; as a result, they get stronger and we get even more stuck in our ways. Through new habits – like yoga – and more helpful ways of thinking and being we can grow and strengthen new pathways. This is known as neuroplasticity, which means our brains are adaptable. We no longer need the old habits in quite the same way. So in many ways, the best practice for someone struggling with addiction is one that is done regularly. By now you will also hopefully know that regularly means little if it is not done in a balanced way and with mindful compassion. Yet certain types of pose are particularly helpful in letting us let go of or 'eliminate' old behaviours and habits that no longer serve us.

- **Poses of elimination and letting go**

It is often said that we carry our baggage, our past stories, on our backs. We can help let these go passively – by doing any of the restorative poses on our backs, symbolically allowing the past to seep away into the earth – or actively – by doing strong backbends which can fortify and may bring a sense of 'throwing off' that which is stuck.

Another way of eliminating is, of course, via the more prosaic and practical one – the digestive system. Much current research tells us that the gut is the second brain, that gut health underpins so much of general health and that both brains – the one in the gut and the one in the head – need to be in good health to communicate better. Yogically, the gut can be targeted in two ways:

- Squatting poses such as *utkatasana* (chair) or *malasana* (garland) help bring the energy downwards and encourage thoughts and feelings of releasing and letting drop.

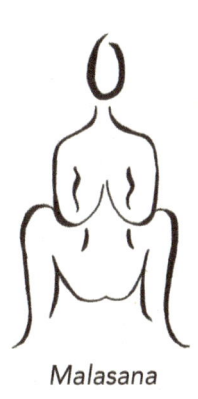

Malasana

- Twisting poses – whether relatively simple ones like *ardha matsyendrasana* (half-lord of the fishes) or the more challenging such as *parvritta trikkonasana* (revolved triangle) – encourage our feelings and thoughts to turn to letting go of stagnant energy. Both squats and twists compress then release both the ascending and descending colons in turn, so encouraging elimination of a more physical kind as well.

- *Tarasana* (star pose) has us bowing the head to the feet – a metaphor about accepting that your head doesn't always know best.

- **Kapalabhati pranayama**

The translation of this is 'shining skull breath', so powerful are its reputed cleansing properties. It pumps out old, stagnant breath from deep in the lungs and is thought to move and expel stale thoughts and energy. It involves using the lower transverse abdominals – strengthening these key core muscles as it does so – to forcefully push out the breath through the nostrils. This rapid exhalation lowers carbon dioxide levels and increases oxygen. When the ratios are reversed we are more easily tipped into a panicky response, so this is a centring breath. The stimulation of the abdominal organs also supports digestive health – and therefore our ability to eliminate, in the most fundamental way, that which is not needed.

Just as in yoga, so in therapy. Here too we think about what we need to let go of, what is weighing us down – whether that be something in the present, or from the past, or our ingrained ways of thinking.

Of course, we need to acknowledge, talk about and learn from the past and how it has contributed to making us who we are. Yet it is also important to know when to put down that burden, to let it go, see it for what it is – something that has passed. It informs you, is part of you, but it doesn't have to define you. You can change and let go of whatever is no longer helpful.

We've spent a lot of time looking at how unhelpful binaries are, and it can be just as easy to fall into binary polarised thinking when it comes to acknowledging your past. Some of us are trapped there, always thinking about how wronged we were, how unfair life has been, how we will never get over it. Others refuse to acknowledge their past, never look behind, so can never learn from past mistakes, never see how much they are being controlled by old habits that no longer serve. The truth, as always, lies somewhere in between. Life is not actually all that linear. It's not one steady path; it loops and it swirls and it spirals and sometimes we find ourselves retracing our steps. Sometimes that's helpful, sometimes it's not. There are times when it's useful to look back and acknowledge what we went through, to be compassionate towards what our younger self had to go through. At other times we need to draw on what the adversity taught us and focus on all the good things, all the strength and knowledge we've gained from them. Sometimes we need to understand that the future can be what we make of it and we don't need to dwell on what has gone. None of these are absolutes; they are relative to the situation and to the person and can all exist simultaneously.

Your addiction or habit does not have to control you. As Kyle's story tells us, it's not about the drugs – it's about acknowledging the pain and the missed connections that they were trying to mask. He found the strength to surrender to this truth and he re-found himself through yoga.

Yoga Saved My Life
Kyle Ely Goldstein

I was powerless over my addiction.

It wasn't about the drugs. Let me say that again, IT WASN'T ABOUT THE DRUGS. They were only a symptom of the bigger problem, which was me.

My inability to deal with life on life's terms was the problem. My inability to deal with my feelings was the problem. My inability to feel comfortable in my own skin, to be confident in who I was and respect myself was the problem.

Throughout the years, I tried so many different things, which are life-savers for so many people. But there was only one thing that completely changed my life, opened my eyes and allowed me to dig deep into my subconscious and rediscover myself. And that was yoga.

It's taught me how to be humble. Humility calls upon us to question ourselves, our motives and actions. In this way, it teaches integrity and honesty. It allows us to remember that practice is just that: practice. It is not about distinguishing ourselves by performing virtuosic postures.

It's taught me how to be grateful. I take that off my mat into my life every day.

From the bottom of my heart, Thank You Yoga.

Widening the Window of Tolerance

The window of tolerance refers to the state of arousal in which we function optimally. Within certain parameters we can cope pretty well with strong emotions. We feel them – anger, sadness, shame, for instance – but we cope with them in a relatively well-mediated way. Our brains can register the fact that we are struggling, but can take steps to act in a way that helps to bring us back to a more balanced place – we talk to friends, we cry, we write an angry letter, we go for a walk, do yoga – whatever we know will help us feel better. However, sometimes we feel so overwhelmed by what have become unmanageable emotions that we go beyond what is tolerable, our brains feel flooded and our responses are no longer within the realm of our conscious, rational control.

Some of us have a very broad window of tolerance and can cope with a lot of stress and emotional triggers, while some of us – and this can be due to a large number of varied reasons – have a narrow window of tolerance and are more easily pushed out of this 'comfort zone', even by things that to the outside eye might not seem like such a big deal.

Once we are pushed beyond our window of tolerance our responses become unregulated, unmediated as they are by the thinking brain. The body's physiological response steps in, unleashing emotions that can feel completely overwhelming, too painful and frightening to cope with. It is often this terror that pushes us towards addictions that can feel – in the moment – as though they are the only way of taking the pain of those toxic feelings away. What can then happen is that even the unconscious fear that we might get pushed towards the edges of the window leads to us taking the drink, drugs or other mechanisms we rely on, in order to stay 'safe'.

Some of us find ourselves being pushed out of the upper level of the window of tolerance into hyper-arousal responses such as fight or flight. This often leads us to try to numb the agitation with the anaesthetising qualities that come from overeating, taking drugs, or the fake security we get from buying items that make us feel safe – more clothes or things for the house.

Others among us find that terror pushes us out of the window of tolerance in a downward direction to the hypo-arousal states of numbness, depression and collapse. Again, we try to mitigate the awfulness of these feelings in whatever ways have worked for us in the past – perhaps with more uplifting drugs like cocaine or alcohol.

The myriad ways in which we self-medicate ourselves out of overwhelming toxic emotions are unique to us and take many forms. But what they have in common is that they are all illusory and short-term fixes. They work – sometimes – in the immediacy of the moment but very soon become part of the problem themselves. Over time, they actually lead to a narrowing of the window because even the thought of the emotions makes us so fearful it becomes enough to tip us over the edge. We become unable to tolerate any uncomfortable feelings whatsoever and smaller and smaller discomforts push us out.

The long-term answer is to work to expand the window of tolerance so that fewer things push us beyond the comfort of its boundaries into unhealthy addictive means of coping. Yoga uses the movement of the body to calm the mind. A repeated regular practice will therefore, over time help to broaden the window of tolerance. If what felt unmanageable has become manageable – tolerable – we have fewer reasons to need artificial help.

People will do anything, no matter how absurd, to avoid facing their own souls.

Carl Jung

CHAPTER SEVENTEEN

The Trauma Response

Trauma can narrow the window of tolerance considerably. It can develop from a one-off event such as a car accident, rape, kidnap or witnessing a loved one die. It can also be the result of an accumulation of events over many years – such as war or imprisonment – and it can be caused by growing up in an environment of neglect or abuse.

Trauma describes your response to an event, not the event itself. It is your body reacting in the instinctive way that it needs to in order to save your life by triggering the fight/flight/freeze response. This affects your whole being – nervous system, brain, breathing, muscles, memory. Consequently, there is an effect on your emotions, your behaviour, your ability to adapt and change and your ability to self-regulate. It is a necessary and useful response to threat to life (which can take many forms, not merely the most obvious – for example, someone trapped in an abusive home life may not be literally endangered, but it can feel as though this is the case). However, what is a useful and life-saving response in the moment of threat is sometimes not turned off even once the danger has passed. This can result in post-traumatic stress (PTS).

How PTS Manifests

PTS symptoms fall into three categories: hyper (which corresponds to the fight response), avoidance (flight) and hypo (freeze or flop). Many PTS sufferers exhibit elements of all three responses, some only one or two.

- Hyper responses can manifest as phobias, flashbacks, hypervigilance, insomnia, nightmares, anxiety, panic attacks, a heightened startle response and mood swings, especially rage, even violence.
- Avoidance responses include agoraphobia, avoiding seeing certain people or things or going to certain places, not allowing in certain thoughts and feelings, OCD, amnesia and anaesthetising activities such as drink and drugs or indulging in obsessive workaholism, social media scrolling, overeating or any other addictive behaviours used to prevent feeling authentic emotion.
- Hypo responses include a numbness in either or both body and mind, dissociation, depression, suicidal thoughts, existential angst, guilt, illness and over-compliance.

If you are suffering from any or a combination of these symptoms, then your ability to function normally is going to be affected, even if on the surface you may look to the outside world (often to yourself as well) as though you are fully functioning, 'successful' even.

Treating Trauma Via the Body

Research has for a long time suggested that treating PTS with regular talking therapy has only limited success. PTS is a physiological

The Trauma Response

response (see page 194) so it is a physical resetting that is needed. The limbic, survival-focused, reactive emotions have split off from the neo-cortex and are unable to take on board its thinking, rational, verbal functions, so appealing verbally to this split-off part is not getting to the heart of the problem. This lack of integration also means that a traumatic event, rather than being remembered and relegated to one's past as it would normally, continues to intrude on the trauma sufferer's life in visual, auditory and other somatic, tangible ways, causing them to relive the life-threatening experience(s) over and over; mind and body reacting as though they are still happening.

Trying to manage these symptoms takes a lot of effort and energy and it can start to rule your life. You may start to fear not just the trauma but your own reaction to it. It becomes a vicious circle:

trigger—response—fear of symptom—symptom becomes new trigger

Each successive turn of this toxic merry-go-round increases stress hormones and decreases your ability to process them healthily.

While the neo-cortex has little sway over the limbic brain, it too is affected by trauma. MRI scans show visible damage to its language centres. This leads to some deactivation in these areas that can continue for years after the event. And if the brain's language centre has been compromised AND parts of the brain are not communicating with each other, talk therapy is clearly going to have limited success; even if we can understand rationally *why* we react as we do, that won't necessarily change how terrified or paralysed we feel, nor can we change those reactions merely by thinking about it. The brain alone cannot abolish bodily memories of terror and threat, so therapists are increasingly incorporating less verbal methods of working with trauma – approaches such as EMDR (Eye Movement Desensitisation and Reprocessing) and EFT (Emotional Freedom Techniques). And, of course, yoga. When the verbal isn't available, yoga gives us the option to instead work directly with the body. And this is useful because in trauma, despite parts of the brain not communicating properly, the lines of communication and influence ARE still open between the emotional brain and the body.

The trauma may have become locked in the nervous system and the muscles in contrasting ways – the fight-or-flight activation may have led to a heightened sense of tension, muscles at the ready to spring into action, or the freeze response may have numbed the body against the pain and stored memories of powerlessness. Either way, the body can feel like it has a life of its own, one you have no control over.

So you need a yoga practice that helps you regain a sense of control. And that starts with feeling safe.

Yoga can help you find a healthier way to contact and listen to the body without it feeling overwhelming, but in order to do so it has to confront a difficult paradox: you need to use the body – the home of the trauma – to cure the trauma. If you are severely traumatised, even the most compassionate of practices can be triggering, or can alternatively just push you deeper into the sort of behaviour that you are trying to change. If this is you, then Trauma Sensitive Yoga could be worth considering.

- **Trauma Sensitive Yoga (TSY)**

Bessel van der Kolk is one of the foremost trauma psychotherapists and academics in the world. The title of his book *The Body Keeps the Score* sums up just how embedded is trauma in the physical bodies of those who have experienced it. His years of research alongside yoga teacher Dave Emerson, culminated in a radical new approach to yoga, devised specifically to work with people whose traumatic experiences have led them to become dissociated from their bodies.

TSY is differentiated from more common forms of yoga by, among other things, the very careful attention that it pays to language and its focus on 'suggesting' as opposed to 'instructing', so that a trauma survivor can take control of their own decisions, and slowly learn to reacquaint themselves with a body that has felt at best alienated, at worst like an enemy. In fact, with TSY I'd *suggest* even putting the word 'yoga' out of your mind. It is more like a relationship-building exercise with a body from which you have been estranged.

You need a teacher qualified in Trauma Sensitive Yoga to guide you, but here is a flavour of what such a class might sound like:

- If you are willing, you can take the option of practising seated in a chair.
- If you are willing, you can notice how the chair feels beneath your sitting bones, beneath your thighs, your ankles, wherever your body is in contact with it. Can you feel this contact? If not, don't worry, just notice that you don't feel much.
- If you are willing [notice how often phrases about willingness occur; it's a reminder that consent is not a one-off thing and that it can change at any time], you can try to promote some sensation by maybe tapping or rubbing your feet against the floor, or lifting and lowering them.
- If you're willing, maybe try swaying from side to side to locate your sitting bones, or lifting and lowering your hands from

your thighs. Try anything you like to make contact and feel a sensation. And if everything still feels numb and uncontactable, then notice that without judgement too.
- Throughout, try accepting each invitation to move as just that – an invitation, not a command. You can choose whether to do it or not; you are in control.
- Now invite yourself, if you are willing, to raise your arms out to the sides. Notice how that feels. Where do you feel the movement? Is it only in the arms or do you also feel movement or changes in other parts of your body as your arms move? Can your hands feel the sensation of a breeze as they pass through the air? Does it feel different if you stretch the fingers wide or ball your hands into fists? Do your shoulders move more or differently the higher the arms rise? Can you still feel the support of the floor or chair beneath your sitting bones and thighs? As you lower the arms again, notice if that changes anything. Do you prefer the feeling of lifting, or the feeling of dropping?

From these few examples you can see how by focusing on smaller, relatively simple movements you have the chance to check in and notice how many different elements go into something as everyday as lifting your arms in the air.

When you realise you can change the way you feel with different movements and intensities, you start to use your body as a resource, allowing it to help not hinder you regain control. Then your body's responses will no longer be things that just happen to you, but become things you can influence.

The theory behind TSY is that it aims to slowly introduce you to four stages of contact with yourself:

The Trauma Response

First, by 'noticing' the different parts, you are able to <u>reclaim</u> this body from which you have become so disconnected.

Second, by 'checking in' and seeing whether even the tiniest of everyday movements feel acceptable, you are setting about <u>befriending</u> your body, developing a relationship with it, becoming interested in it, establishing trust.

Third, you start to gain a sense of <u>agency</u> – so important if your trauma has rendered you powerless. TSY reveals to you that you can change the way you feel with different movements, with altering the intensity – the effort, or ease – of what you do and the attitude with which you do it. You learn how much you need to put in. It can be very empowering to know that you have agency over your own life, choices and directions.

Fourth, in practising making <u>choices</u>, you find <u>purpose</u>. You come to realise that you can make decisions about what feels right to you. Not only that, but those choices are based on bodily experience, which puts you back in charge. You come to learn cause and effect – if I move this muscle in this way, this is the result. You are purposefully making that intensity and purposefully releasing it. You are controlling what you do.

Perhaps most importantly of all, though, TSY allows you to experience what it is like to feel safe within your body. All the trauma research is clear – if you re-provoke old fears, you re-harden old defences, and old habits re-emerge. So always remember the yogic principle of practising with *ahimsa*, with self-compassion, and your body can again start to feel like a friend. Whether you have PTS severely, mildly or not at all, practising with these principles in mind will lead to a more attentive and respectful relationship with your body.

Yoga Saved My Life
Natalie Terhaar (Lindner)

My fiancé was diagnosed with squamous cell carcinoma of the oral tongue on Thanksgiving 2011.

Just six gruelling months after his diagnosis, with me as his primary caretaker, he passed away. I held his memorial service on my thirtieth birthday. As all my friends were getting married and having babies, I was a 'widow', living at my parents' house, having to start my life completely over.

I instinctively wanted to curl inwards and disappear. I became numb. I was told that I had PTSD from what I had witnessed throughout his illness. I went to my first power yoga class and remember sobbing during *savasana*. I walked out and knew this was exactly what I needed. Yoga saved my life.

My anxiety and fears had been pushed to the max and I had lost control. Yoga was a way to push myself on my own terms.

They say that yoga releases physical memory and I believe that with every sweat drop, a negative memory faded.

The message was to move on and to not feel guilty about it, to take care of myself and to recognise how strong I was. There is hope and there is always yoga.

The Physiology of Trauma

When we believe our lives are in danger, we revert to ancient methods of saving ourselves. In human prehistory, danger was often very literally life-threatening – it took the form of,

The Trauma Response

say, a snake or a lion. And the action needed when faced with one of these was – still is – whatever will minimise the risk: fight, flight or freeze.

When survival is at stake, the terror is too much for the neo-cortex, the newer, thinking part of the brain, to process. We need action not thought, for which the older part – the instinctive limbic brain – is primed. This is the part of the brain which can respond to danger immediately, activating us physiologically.

The limbic brain tells the body to unleash the action hormones, adrenaline and cortisol. These catapult us into extreme sympathetic nervous system domination – the heart beats faster, blood pumps faster, we start sweating in order to cool our internal organs, we take in more oxygen. All these things prime our muscles for action and shut down non-essential functions like digestion or the need for sleep or even our ability to empathise or think rationally. Every part of the body is poised and ready to fight or flee, or in even more extreme circumstances, which I'll come to in a moment, it causes us to freeze instead.

Once we have dealt with the threat, the body should reset and return to normal. The neo-cortex can come back online and we can think clearly again.

It's a great and life-saving response and one which we couldn't do without. But it comes with issues attached, not least that the reset doesn't always happen quickly enough, meaning these dramatic responses continue long beyond when they are actually necessary.

Another problem with it is that the nervous system responds in the same way to both emotional and physical threats. This can make us very reactive to situations that aren't life-threatening on a physical level, but appear so on an emotional one – losing your job, losing your partner, feeling trapped in an abusive relationship, to name but a few possibilities.

Then there is the issue that the pace and stresses of the modern world can mean that the limbic brain becomes oversensitive, endlessly feels threatened and so constantly sends the message to pump out even more of those adrenaline and cortisol hormones. While these are useful for the short term need to fight or flee, if they hang around too long they become destructive and cause chronic stress or post-traumatic stress. The more sensitive the system becomes, the more false alarms we receive, creating a vicious circle. Our body no longer really knows how not to be primed for action.

When we can neither fight nor flee, we freeze instead. In freezing, our dorsal vagal nerve shuts down the body and we dissociate or feel paralysed.

From an evolutionary point of view, this will either make us look to our predator as though we are already dead, meaning they wander off, disappointed, and we escape; or, if not, the freezing provides an anaesthetising effect that means the pain is somewhat numbed. So freezing is, in fact, the most extreme of all the parts of this response; we call on it only if all else fails and it seems that it's probably all over for us.

In the modern world this manifests as paralysis or immobilisation – hence, for instance, why rape victims often do not and cannot fight back as they are sometimes callously exhorted to do. In fact, there is a whole new level of understanding of this freeze response that has been

developed over more recent years. It involves more F
words – words like Friend, Fawn, Faint and Flop. Women
and children's physiology often means they do not have as
many fight-or-flight options available, so other strategies
need to be employed; to immobilise and 'play dead' is just
one – they can also try to appease and empathise with the
aggressor. Trying not to provoke more extreme anger might
be the best and only survival response available. This might
manifest as befriending them or even fawning over them,
which is a good idea given their limited options for fight or
flight.

Physiologically, and the other reason that it is the last-chance-saloon option, freezing takes an even greater toll on our bodies than fighting or fleeing. Essentially, in freeze mode we crash our cortisol- and adrenaline-filled bodies into such severe parasympathetic dominance that everything stops almost-dead. The cost of this paradoxical messaging to our bodies is huge.

In Chapter Six we looked at the wandering vagus nerve, which covers such huge distances, insinuates itself into so many of our vital organs and is so important in communicating across our bodymind.

The dorsal branch of it, as mentioned above, can shut us down, but remember that the other branch, the ventral vagal, can actually mitigate the trauma response. Polyvagal theory tells us that the nervous system's response to threat is not as binary as we once thought. We are, in fact, not just reliant on either the fight/flight or the freeze options. If our ventral vagal nerve has been suitably nurtured and is sufficiently well-toned, then it can provide a more sophisticated 'first resort' option that we can turn to without have to reach for fight or flight so quickly.

In survival mode we are primed to only engage with another person in the sense of lashing out, running away or collapsing/freezing/fawning in response to them. Healthy vagal tone increases our social engagement system and improves relationships, increasing our ability to allow others in, bond and feel empathy and so we are less likely to have to revert to the more extreme survival responses and the trauma response is less easily triggered.

So how do we go about cultivating better vagal toning? Well, therapy helps us in all the ways we've been discussing – by providing a safe space in which we can discover and reveal our vulnerabilities and so learn that threat doesn't always need to result from such close connection. Yoga also provides a safe container for exploration of vulnerabilities and promotes trust. The close attention to the nervous system we are cultivating allows us to spot when we are moving from homeostasis and gives us the tools to rectify this using breath and movement.

Yoga Saved My Life
Ashlee Mcdougall

I was born with cystic fibrosis – a genetic and potentially fatal lung disease – and I wasn't expected to live past eighteen.

My childhood was filled with numerous traumatising procedures and hospitalisations – and back then trauma wasn't widely discussed.

The Trauma Response

I found yoga at a time when I was moving through life unaware of past trauma and reacting accordingly. I didn't understand that stuck energy manifested in my addictive behaviours, extreme emotions, anxiety and disordered eating habits. I genuinely thought that my behaviours and actions were normal and that life was supposed to feel so overwhelming.

It wasn't until I went to a yoga training and had a PTSD flashback in the middle of a yin class that I began to understand that feeling constantly overwhelmed is a sign of trapped energy.

Since then, I have spent years studying how yoga can help facilitate healing by bringing awareness to past hurt (trauma), repairing energy channels and creating a safe space to calm my overwhelmed nervous system.

Yoga gave me the tools to live with intention and mindfulness and helped me to stop living in reactivity.

Healing is a lifelong process and I'm blessed to have found this path.

The ache for home lives in all of us, the safe place where we can go as we are and not be questioned.

Maya Angelou

CHAPTER EIGHTEEN

Is There Anybody Out There?

Yoga Saved My Life
Felicity

I was abused when I was a little girl and I felt abandoned, hurt and lost.

Today I can say that all I have gone through made me the beautiful being I am, not alone any more, because I am surrounded by love, peace and happiness. I see myself in most of the beings I meet in my everyday life.

Before yoga I was insecure, in my body, mind and spirit. I didn't know who I was, always looking for answers; then I discovered that answers weren't needed. I knew that everything is perfect as it is.

I am happy to be vulnerable, I am happy to be a woman, feeling a real woman maybe for the first time in my life!

We are not alone, no one is… We may feel lonely but that is caused by disconnection.

Community, Mother Nature and your freedom are the keys to your connection and grounding.

Is There Anybody Out There?

> No need to hide; we are all on this journey together, so let's row this boat together. Face your fears, take the bad with the good and appreciate the little things.
>
> Namaste.

Loneliness has reached pandemic proportions, with half of all British adults admitting to often feeling deeply lonely.[42] Quite apart from what a painful emotion it is to feel, we now also know that loneliness has very real and life-limiting health risks attached.[43]

Bowlby's attachment theory has shown us that we come into this world primed for connection, that we are born to be sociable, that our survival depends on it. Neuroscience has shown how our brains are wired to connect, and that when that goes awry our very brain chemistry is affected, making us more vulnerable to defensiveness, trauma and addictions in later life – all things that further deepen our disconnection from others. Polyvagal theory has shown that deep connection to others is crucial for self-regulation and soothing.

And yet so many of us are lonely. It seems to be a particularly modern, and Western, problem. Our society values and rewards self-serving behaviour and puts on us the expectation that we should be independent. Its measures of 'success' are limited to the financial, material and status-dependent. At the same time, it stokes our shame around loneliness, forcing us to put on masks and identities to cover up what is seen as the indignity or embarrassment of that disconnect. Society tells us to hide our more authentic selves with all their flaws and vulnerabilities, even though these are the very things that would enable us to develop better, more honest relationships with all the other flawed and vulnerable people out there. All this secrecy, shame and misaligned priorities can mean that sometimes our drive for independence, money and status leads to loneliness. This can very often be the motivating force sending someone into therapy – a recognition of loneliness and a need to learn how to reconnect.

Much of what we have looked at so far has been concerned with withdrawing from the need for the approval of others and becoming surer of ourselves. This is important, of course, but we shouldn't think that our need for inner surety and strength means we don't also need others. Just as much as therapy and yoga help us locate those stronger inner selves, so too do they reveal how necessary and enriching connection can be. Yet for some of us that idea of connection can lead us to fear we will lose all sense of ourselves, that we may just merge into another and be subsumed by them.

Individuality and Merging

Is it possible to retain a strong sense of individuality while also connecting deeply with another? Psychoanalyst Heinz Kohut developed what has come to be known as self-psychology.[44] He recognised that a strong sense of self comes about from being adequately mirrored by and feeling a kinship with another. Only by feeling deeply connected can we feel truly all right when alone, as we are able to carry a representation of the other within.

We have seen that seeming opposites like strength and vulnerability are not mutually exclusive, and, in the same way, that mind and body, thoughts and feelings can all be embraced as equal partners, not adversaries. Two sides of the same coin. In the same way, we can find our independence yet still need others.

Let's look at the idea internally first. As individuals, every day, in every interaction, we embody our own complexity. We move to

Is There Anybody Out There?

and fro between our different selves, from one part to the whole, and back again, which can occasionally seem confusing, contradictory even. We compartmentalise and then we integrate. Here's one way of looking at it. I am both a therapist and a yoga teacher but I can – to some extent – isolate those different roles I inhabit. I can talk and interact from both individual perspectives – my therapy clients don't necessarily know that I am a yoga teacher, nor my yoga students that I am a therapist. Yet I am a different yoga teacher to the one I would be if I weren't also a therapist – such is the integration of that part of me into the other. And I am a different therapist to the one I would be if I weren't also a yoga teacher. In no real way can I remove all that I know and have become from one role and solely inhabit the other without cross-contamination (hopefully in a productive way). Just because we experience things as separate and can see them working individually does not mean they actually are separate, or that they don't need each other. Think about the spine, our literal and metaphorical backbone; if it doesn't work as well as it could, every part of the body is affected. And within the spine, each vertebra has to be individually healthy and work independently, but that means nothing if it doesn't work overall as part of the team, the whole spine.

Externally, this tension manifests in our relationships, where we need to work to find the balance between individuality and togetherness, both of which we need. When apart we carry the representation of our loved one with us, so we are never really alone. When together we need to also keep a sense of our individuality so as not to merge and lose ourselves. We need to emotionally connect with someone without losing the autonomy of our own emotional functioning.

If you are lonely, it can be hard to feel any sense of togetherness or connection to anyone. But once again, the lessons of yoga can help us find connection. Yoga is a practice of continual separating and joining, of isolating and integrating. What am I on about? Let's look at this notion via postures, principles and *pranayama*.

- **Supta padangusthasana**

Yoga is a process of unifying but at the same time it asks us to separate and individuate. We separate in order to connect. Through our bodies we come to understand that each limb, each muscle, each vertebra, each cell is an individual that works alone, but also works within the system. Let's look at some of the elements of *supta padangusthasana* (reclining hand-to-big-toe pose) as an example of how we move from the part to the whole and back again.

- This pose starts with you lying on your back with one leg up in the air. Try taking your awareness into the foot that's in the air and play with the sensations there. For instance, you could crunch your toes together into a tight 'fist', then stretch them wide apart. In doing this you might experience how your toes can act together or separately, and also see that the foot is separate to the rest of the leg which can remain still while you move the foot. And you see how this too is made up of separate parts, which all respond differently to these mini-movements. Each toe may feel different, the arch of the foot may feel different, the inside of the heel, the outside edge. Notice how your foot responds to the attention lavished on it, starts to wake up. Does it perhaps feel cold, warm, pleasant or a bit achy? Tight? Numb?
- What if you flex the foot? You may feel how the ankle now gets involved. Pay attention to its character and how it feels. Let your attention roam further and feel how that small action has woken up the whole of the back of the leg. The hamstring is being stretched and awareness can travel along it. Notice all the

sensations there, way down into the insertion point at the pelvis, even though that's far away from the foot that is doing the movement. There are knock-on effects to the smallest change. Be simultaneously more aware of the individuality of your foot, and of how it connects to the pelvis via the full length of the leg.
- What if you point your toes? You may notice how the front of the leg now wakes up as the quadriceps muscle in the thigh switches from contracting to an extended position. Keep this careful attention going as you continue the pose. Or indeed any pose. At each stage you can feel how by emphasising the small, you affect the large. A butterfly flaps its wings on one side of the world and a storm brews on the other. All is connected. Everything is hitched to something else. Pay attention to the micro, and you can see how you are affecting the macro. This works within our bodies and within our relationships.

- **Work with symmetry. And with asymmetry.**

Many postures work alternately on each side of the body, thus allowing you to see, and more importantly to feel, the differences between them. You learn which side is tighter, which more accessible, all of your body's anomalies. You get to see that as you work each part, you simultaneously work the whole. You learn that you need to treat different parts differently, and by doing so you absorb the lessons of connection and individuality; that you can honour and admire difference while still remaining open to communication. As a whole you can be more than the sum of your parts.

Take *supta padangusthasana*, from above. Once you have done the full pose on one leg, try lying flat in *savasana* (corpse or relaxation pose) and feel into the side of the body that you've been exploring. How warm is it, how soft, how long is the leg that was in the air, how alive is it; what other qualities or sensations do you notice? Now switch your attention to the side you haven't explored and see what you find there. You will likely notice differences; one that is usually quite easy to feel (and that many people do feel slightly freaked out about) is the sense that the leg you've worked on is much longer than the other.

Other differences exist in all sorts of less obvious ways. By refining your awareness you can bring these anomalies and discrepancies more and more into consciousness, just as in therapy you may start by looking at a very marked concern – let's say loneliness, to use this chapter's subject – and with careful, compassionate exploration you can see all the myriad micro-patterns and habits that may be contributing and how by changing one or two small, ingrained things, something larger can start to occur.

Yoga provides us with a whole raft of asymmetrical postures that ask us to focus on one side at a time and so teach us what independence feels like. Yoga's principles of sequencing generally then ask us to counterbalance these with symmetrical poses, which means we experience the contrast: unity and integration. As always, neither is better or worse, good or bad; all are necessary.

• Cross-lateral poses

Neuroscience tells us that the two hemispheres of the brain similarly work both separately and together.[45] Each has its speciality – the right brain tends more to the artistic and instinctive, while the left more towards the practical and logical – but neither works in isolation and each affects the other. Promoting neural growth and improving the lines of communication between the two provides a richness of knowledge and experience that neither could achieve alone.

Cross-lateral postures – meaning those which involve crossing the midline of the body – help promote this growth and communication. There are many, many poses in this category. A relatively simple one is *dandayamana bharmanasana* or balancing table pose. This has you on all fours, stretching out your right arm and reaching forwards, while also reaching your left leg backwards. You can then curl elbow in towards knee to touch as they reach each other at your midline, which really lets your brain – as well as your body – understand integration in a very practical way. Physical coordination, as called on in this pose, improves cognitive coordination. It also promotes proprioception – our awareness of ourselves in space – which increases awareness of where we are in relation to others. Off the yoga mat, this can help with socialisation.

More complex postures for exploring this principle include any of the twisted standing balances – for instance, *parivrtta ardha chandrasana* (revolved half-moon) or *garudasana* (eagle).

- **Nadi shodhana pranayama**

In English this gets translated as alternate nostril breathing. *Nadi shodhana* is in many ways the breathing equivalent of a crosslateral asana. It involves using the fingers to block first one nostril, then the other in turn – breathing in and out through one at a time, alternating between nostrils – and is considered to be balancing and stress-reducing.

We all, naturally and unconsciously, alternate our breathing through first one nostril, then the other in a roughly two-hour cycle. When one nostril is dominant, its blood vessels and other structures are engorged with blood and active, and the other has the chance to decongest and rejuvenate.

Physiologically, the right nostril stimulates the sympathetic nervous system, promoting activity; the left the parasympathetic nervous system, aiding relaxation.[46] Yogic philosophy also believes the two nostrils represent energy channels in the body. We have *ida nadi* on the left and *pingala nadi* on the right. Practising *nadi shodhana* actively balances the duration of the domination of each nostril, harmonising the nervous system, or in yogic terms, strengthening the middle energy channel – *sushumna nadi*.

Again, this is a practice that allows us to experience how separation and focus on one side can ultimately promote better integration of the whole.

Community

Coming to understand how connected we all are, how profoundly a seemingly small action can affect others, may reduce feelings of isolation and make you feel more engaged, part of a bigger picture.

Practically speaking too, yoga can help combat loneliness, by providing a warm and inclusive community. Every story in this book in some way expresses a feeling of togetherness, of 'coming home'.

You can also be part of a community in person at your local yoga studio. Wherever you practise, you can turn up on your mat safe in the knowledge that the person next to you (whatever they seem to be doing on the outside) is sharing a version of the suffering and learning and enjoying and relaxing that you too are experiencing as you practise together. We are not so different. Quite the opposite, in fact – as you find yourself attuning to others, you may be able to be with them in a more meaningful, reciprocal way. Remember everything we have learned about vulnerability and how it contributes to deeper, more worthwhile connections? Your yoga practice has been working on increasing your compassion which will enable you to open more and better connect to others.

The more integrated we can become, the more internally harmonious in mind and body, the more integrated and harmonious we will be with others.

Is There Anybody Out There?

Yoga Saved My Life
Kim Ludbrook

I am a photojournalist and have covered every aspect of the human condition through the viewfinder of my camera, including the invasion of Iraq in 2003, the 2011 civil war in Libya, the 2004 civil war in Liberia, the aftermath of the Asian tsunami, a coup d'état in Madagascar and thousands of violent/angry protests and failed elections in Africa.

The tens of thousands of images I shot have been imprinted in my mind and soul alongside horrific sounds/smells/tastes/sights and for years I unconsciously tried to hide those experiences through alcohol abuse, riding with a motorcycle gang and living, in retrospect, a very unconscious life.

Then overnight, ten years ago, my soul spoke and I realised I needed an intervention.

Guided meditation helped me process the countless traumatic events I had lived through.

Through meditation came my love affair with yoga.

I am SO grateful for my experiences on the front lines because they ultimately led to my spiritual awakening and to a more conscious life.

We are like islands in the sea, separate on the surface but connected in the deep.

William James

CHAPTER NINETEEN

Shall We Dance?

Yoga Saved My Life
Joey Scherr

My husband and I were ready to start a family and I followed him and his job to Saudi Arabia, where things quickly went downhill. I developed depression, anxiety attacks, acne, an eating disorder and was eventually diagnosed with PCOS. My ovaries were covered in cysts and doctors told me it was unlikely I would ever have children.

The only way I could pause my racing mind was to lose myself in my yoga practice. The routine and dedication gave me something to focus on.

I was teaching yoga on the compound where we lived. I poured my heart and soul into helping my students grow. It felt like the only thing I could get right. As my body got stronger, I built up the mental strength to leave. My husband wouldn't come with me so I left everything.

Today I have built a life around yoga. I specialise in empowering women, running Shakti women's circles, pre- and post-natal yoga, hypnobirthing and offering yoga to female refugees.

Shall We Dance?

> My body has healed beyond recognition and I hope to one day have a family. As my physical strength has developed, so has my mental strength, confidence and sense of self. Helping others is something I find deeply nourishing. Yoga started out as an escape from my life and ultimately saved my life.

What the last chapter was really about was negotiating a dance between aloneness and connection. And we all know that for any sort of dance, rhythm is vital. The give and take of a relationship can be what makes or breaks its comfort and success, and it consists of what you do, what you say and what you don't say. All interactions require some sort of dance, some sort of rhythm and some of us are better at it than others.

Nature's elements too are constantly dancing in rhythm – while one gives another takes. As the sun advances the moon retreats, as winter steps back, summer steps forwards, all while high and low tides sway seamlessly and constantly from one to the other. Neuroscientists now know that we too are engaging in a dance of give and take as we communicate with each other at levels out of conscious awareness.[47] One person's nervous system can talk to another's, can influence another's without even a word being spoken.

Most of us learn this interactive dance as infants. The way a parent and baby communicate through sound, touch and facial expressions enables an infant to self-regulate via the parent's regulation, and it learns how to comfortably attune to others.[48]

Some of us, due to mis-attuned caregivers, never learned this as babies but are able to discover better ways of tuning in to others through the intimacy of the psychotherapeutic relationship. Yoga too allows us to find a co-created rhythm. By following the movement and the breath of the teacher and the rest of the class we can experience what being in rhythm and sync with another person feels like without words. It gives a taste of the synchronicity of moving together that we may have missed out on in early life. This rhythmical attunement facilitates other kinds of attunement experience, allowing for deeper and more meaningful relationships.

Yoga also helps us tune in to and align with life's ebb and flow as we are constantly using little micromovements to adjust to and within each posture. Even when we are still, the breath continues to move, just as the surface of a lake dances almost imperceptibly even on the calmest days. This happens throughout each posture and each transition between them, but as always I am going to suggest a couple of ways of practising that might help this notion feel more embodied.

- **Moving in *vinyasa*/stillness in *nidra***

These first suggestions may seem contradictory on the surface, but are really just two expressions of complementary tides flowing in and out, high to low.

Vinyasa or flow yoga is energising and active. It doesn't tend to linger in each asana. It is less about holding, aligning and observing than it is about transitioning, keeping the postures flowing one into the other. We sometimes have a tendency to think the 'final' posture, held still, is the point. And sometimes it is. But try making the transitions between each posture your focus instead; you will have a different sort of experience. And a valuable one; you will see how it can be not just about the end point or the 'achievement' but about the journey. Rather than thinking anything is ever perfect and finished, it's a lesson in how the journey is ever flowing, ever continuing.

Shall We Dance?

Flowing like this also helps us tune in to our inner fluidity, our inner dance, and – if we are in a group session – we also flow in tune and in time with those around us, viscerally feeling that sense of being part of a fluidly dancing whole.

If *vinyasa* is a high tide at midday in summer, then a low-tide, moonlit winter is yoga *nidra*. This is 'yogic sleep', where your consciousness hovers within that fluid, liminal arena between waking and sleeping. Your supine body is still, just the gentle beats of the heart and the rhythmic lifting and falling waves of breath. Your awareness (generally guided by a teacher's calm voice) softly visits each body part in turn, gently roams across spectrums, imagining first heat then cold, first oceans then deserts, night then day and so on, allowing the dance of opposites to exist and flow together.

There have been many studies into the benefits of yoga *nidra*, and MRIs have demonstrated that the practice has a visible effect on rewiring the brain. *Nidra* has been shown not only to rewire neural circuits, but also to increase levels of dopamine, the pleasure hormone, by 60 per cent.[49]

- **Revisit *adho mukha svanasana***

Downward dog is possibly the most 'visited' asana of all. Barely a class goes by without it featuring multiple times. So why I am focusing on it here?

- Many of us are so familiar with this posture that we stop thinking about it and just do it on automatic pilot – and we've already learned about the perils inherent in that.
- It requires many parts of the body to work together at once; there's barely a bit of us that doesn't need to be engaged, to work in harmony with the other parts.

- Although often described as a resting posture, it may feel to most of us that it requires vast reserves of strength and endurance. It took me about two decades of struggle with this one before I realised that I was indeed finally starting to find it restful. Talk about a lesson in patience and the rewards that can come from perseverance!
- It is a good example of a posture that manages to dance along that tightrope of being both energising and calming at once. Had I been able to embody and make peace with the inherent contradictions in it sooner, realise the need to hold two contrasting truths at once, I would have done a lot less sweating and fighting it. But then again, as we have seen, the only way out is through. I had to learn this the hard way. As a Buddhist saying goes – when we are ready to learn the lesson, the teacher will appear. *Adho mukha svanasana* was my teacher in this, just as other asanas have been my teachers in ways varied, lengthy and often painful, over many years.
- It is a good example of how a seemingly static posture is actually teeming with movement if you dig down into it. For instance, if you focus purely on your legs, you may soon realise that your shoulders have risen towards your neck. So you can move your attention there and bring the shoulders back and down and concentrate on pressing into the ground through the palms. Until you realise these little adjustments mean your feet are now no longer quite as connected as they once were, so you go back and re-ground, and on it goes. The breath continues to flow, the clouds of thought continue to float past, the micro-adjustments continue to happen. The dance continues.
- It is an inversion, and we have seen how inversions literally and otherwise shift our view of ourselves and also of others. Through them we can learn to value diversity and the dance

Shall We Dance?

between people, and to get more in step with those who appear to be dancing to a different rhythm, singing a different tune. Maybe with some micro-adjusting we can find a dance we can all join in with?

Yoga makes a sincere practitioner into an integrated personality. It develops a feeling of oneness between man and nature, between man and man, and between man and his Maker, thus permitting the experience of a feeling of identity with the spirit that pervades all creation.

B.K.S. Iyenger

CHAPTER TWENTY

Dive In

Yoga Saved My Life
Jessica Erb

'Fat bodies can't teach yoga'… I was trapped in that mindset for years.

I'd pushed my poor body to its limit, taking classes to burn, torch, shred, shake the fat off, while also starving it. I triggered a severe hip injury; it left me in chronic pain.

Up until my first class, I thought yoga was boring stretching. I accidentally took an advanced *vinyasa* class for my first go! I saw neighbours lift into headstands and others remain in wide folds. The instructor didn't tell people to go further than they could because 'that's where the magic happens'. She reminded the class to respect what their bodies were saying to them. This was revolutionary! Do something to be kind to my body and not as an act of battle?!

I discovered if I became frustrated, impatient, the more I struggled in poses. Yet, the more I took my time and gave my body positive encouragement, the more I could progress, or just be joyful in whatever variation.

Yoga gave me a way to move my body with kindness. Teaching yoga is a platform to act out against body shame.

Dive In

> I'm a fat girl with a bum hip, but I joyfully do what I can do and accept working on things I cannot do… yet.

Savasana, corpse pose, is a crucial element to our practice. It is the time when we get to stop and absorb the many lessons taught us by the more active poses that precede it. Perhaps we could think of this closing chapter in our journey together as the written version of a *savasana*. A place where we can relax, reflect back on and absorb all that we have experienced together.

In both yoga and therapy we swim in emotionally deep waters, learning to cope with the ebb and flow that comes with that. We all know water can be life-giving and life-destroying, joyful and painful, nurturing and freezing. If you can learn to swim, though, you will be less fearful of its power, more able to make choices as to how you interact with it. Yoga and psychotherapy give you the ability to swim through the ever-changing turbulent ocean of life.

I don't think any of the individuals' stories here suggest that the journey into oneself that yoga can bring about is without challenge. They describe many huge waves that have threatened to dunk them under on multiple occasions. Yet what each and every one of them does so powerfully is celebrate the life-enhancing gains that those challenges bring in their wake, and highlight the skills yoga has given them to help them rise back up to the surface more quickly.

Yoga's Gifts

Yoga helps us to recognise our edge and have the courage and skill to know when to try to transcend it and when to retreat from it.

We become brave enough to move forwards and face whatever unknowns appear, knowing that our fear is understandable and manageable, and that we will not be thrown off course by the unexpected. We won't need to double down on our defences, create a cage to box ourselves into or make ourselves so rigid that we snap. Nor will we collapse into chaos and helplessness without the ability to find our feet, stand our ground, discover a backbone and hold our heads high. We know who we are, have a solid sense of self alongside a strong connection to others and are able to help and be helped.

Yoga shows us a third way, so we can integrate all parts of the brain, old and new, left and right; integrate the bottom-up body-initiated messages with the top-down brain-initiated messages; integrate our explicit and implicit memories, our conscious and our unconscious, our past, present and future; integrate our many selves – the strong, the vulnerable, the achiever, the nurturer. We no longer have to be 'the sort of person who'; instead all selves are invited to the party. We start to make sense to ourselves and, as a result, to others. We can integrate our individual self with others, open ourselves up to relationship. We can dance in rhythm with those others, able to understand that their way of being is not ours, and that that is more than okay – it is enriching. Possibly, we can even think about integrating this world with another, feeling part of a larger, more transcendental whole.

By going off balance we can find our balance. By going upside down we can find the right way up. By finding our strength we can find our softness. By allowing our vulnerability we can find our bravery.

What all of this gives birth to is a more fully rounded narrative in the story of us. It may have hitherto felt like we were living a script written by others. Now we can control the narrative.

Instead of simplistic black and white we have nuance – a full spectrum of colour, a full orchestra of sound, a full complement of senses. An academic psychotherapist called Bromberg describes this another way – he says it is like standing in the spaces between realities, without losing any of them.[50] I'd say it is also being able to appreciate the uniqueness of each individual voice, as well as how it enhances the harmony of the choir.

The honest, moving stories of the individuals in this book have each described all the ways in which yoga has transformed and saved them. For many it was discovering yoga for the first time and being opened up to new ways of being. For others it was about the deepening of an existing practice.

Michelangelo said:

'The sculpture is already complete within the marble block before I start my work. It is already there, I just have to chisel away the superfluous material.'

Just as Michelangelo liberated each of his sculptures from the marble in which it was hidden, yoga gives us a way to similarly dissolve the superfluous stone in which we are trapped by circumstances. Therapy does too. With these twin scaffolding posts in place, we can all find our way through an unpredictable future. We can evolve as psychotherapy and yoga have. We are all works in progress and with yoga to help us we can enjoy watching our story unfold, safe in the knowledge that our hand is on the tiller of a strong and stable boat carrying the resources to ride out the waves of whatever the ocean brings us. Thank you for sailing these seas alongside me. I bid you all farewell on your journey into yoga and into yourselves, but more than that I hope you enjoy the ride.

We can let the circumstances of our lives harden us so that we become increasingly resentful and afraid, or we can let them soften us, and make us kinder. You always have the choice.

Dalai Lama

Bibliography

Aposhyan, S. (2004) *Body-Mind Psychotherapy: Principles, Techniques and Practical Applications*. New York: W. W. Norton and Company.

Armstrong, J., Rishi, K. (2020) *The Bhagavad Gita Comes Alive: A radical translation*. Vancouver: VASA Publishing.

Balasubramaniam, M. et al. (2012) 'Yoga on our Minds: a Systematic Review of Yoga for Neuropsychiatric Disorders'. *Frontiers in Psychiatry*. Pre-published online 12 October 2012. doi: 10.3389/fpsyt.2012.00117

Becker, I. (2008) 'Uses of Yoga in Psychiatry and Medicine'. *Complementary and Alternative Medicine and Psychiatry*, vol 19: 107–42.

Bion, W. R. (1970) *Attention and Interpretation*. London: Tavistock Publications Ltd.

Boadella, D. (1973) *Wilhelm Reich, the Evolution of his Work*. Chicago: Henry Regnery Company.

Boadella, D. (1987) *Lifestreams: An introduction to Biosynthesis*. London: Routledge and Kegan Paul.

Boellinghaus, I., Jones, F. W. and Hutton, J. (2014) 'The Role of Mindfulness and Loving-kindness Meditation in Cultivating Self-compassion and Other-focused Concern in Health Care Professionals'. *Mindfulness* 5, 129–38. doi: 10.1007/s12671-012-0158-6

Bowlby, J. (1969) *Attachment and Loss*. London: Random House.

Bowlby, J. (1988) *A Secure Base*. Abingdon: Routledge.

Brisbon, N. M. and Lowery, G. A. (2011) 'Mindfulness and Levels of Stress: A comparison of beginner and advanced hatha yoga practitioners'. *Journal of Religion and Health*, 50, no.4, 931–41. doi: 10.1007/s10943-009 9305-3

Bromberg, P. M. (1996) 'Standing in the spaces: The multiplicity of self and the psychoanalytic relationship'. *Contemporary Psychoanalysis*, 32(4); 509–35.

Bibliography

Brown, R. P. and Gerbarg, P. L. (2009) 'Yoga Breathing, Meditation and Longevity'. *Annals of the New York Academy of Sciences* 1172, 54–62. doi: 10.1111/j.1749-6632.2009.04394.x

Caldwell, C. and Johnson, R. (2012) 'Research 101 for Body Psychotherapists: Cultivating a Somatically-informed Research Mind'. In Young, C. (2012) *About the Science of Body Psychotherapy.* Galashiels: Body Psychotherapy Publications.

Caplan, M. (2018). *Yoga and Psyche: integrating the paths of yoga and psychology for healing, transformation and joy.* Boulder, Colorado: Sounds True.

Chitty, J. (2013) *Dancing with Yin and Yang: Ancient Wisdom, Modern Psychotherapy and Randolph Stone's Polarity Therapy.* Boulder, Colorado: Redwood Press.

Christopher, J. C. and Maris, J. A. (2010) 'Integrating Mindfulness as Self-care Into Counselling and Psychotherapy Training'. *Counselling and Psychotherapy Research,* 2010, June 10(2): 114–25.

Cope, S. (1999) *Yoga and the Quest for the True Self.* New York: Bantam.

Cope, S. (2003) *Will Yoga and Meditation Really Change my Life?* North Adams: Storey.

Cozolino, L. (2002, 2017) *The Neuroscience of Psychotherapy: Healing the Social Brain.* London: W. W. Norton and Company.

Cozolino, L.(2006, 2014) *The Neuroscience of Human Relationships: Attachment and the Developing Social Brain.* London: W. W. Norton and Company.

Craig, A. D. (2003) 'Interoception: the sense of the physiological condition of the body'. *Current Opinion in Neurobiology,* 13(4), 500–505.

Craig, A. D. (2010) 'The Sentient Self'. *Brain Structure and Function,* 214 (5–6): 563–77.

Dalai Lama, his holiness the and Cutler, H. C (1998), *The Art of Happiness,* London: Hodder and Stoughton.

Dalai Lama, his holiness the and Hopkins, J. (ed. and translator) (2002) *How to Practice.* London: Random House.

Damasio, A. (1994) *Descartes' Error: Emotion, Reason and the Human Brain.* New York: Penguin.

Damasio, A. (1999) *The Feeling of What Happens: Body and Emotion in the Making of Consciousness.* New York: Hartcourt Bruce.

Davidson, R. J. and Kabat-Zinn, J. (2003) 'Alterations in Brain and Immune Function Produced by Mindfulness Meditation'. *Psychosomatic Medicine* 65(4): 564–70.

Devasena, I. and Narhare, P. (2011) 'Effect of yoga on heart rate and blood pressure and its clinical significance'. *International Journal of Biological and Medical Research,* 2011; 2(3): 75–753.

Dunn, R., Callahan, J. L., Swift, J. K. and Ivanovich, M. (2012) 'Effects of Pre-Session Centering For Therapists on Session Presence and Effectiveness'. *Psychotherapy Research.* doi: 10.1080/10503307.2012.731713

Dunn, K. D. (2008) 'A review of the literature examining the physiological processes underlying the therapeutic benefits of Hatha yoga'. *Adv Mind Body Med,* 2008, September 23(3): 10–8.

Eastman-Mueller, H., Wilson, T., Jung, A-K., Kimura, A. and Tarrant, J. (2013) 'iRest Yoga-Nidra on the College Campus: changes in stress, depression, worry and mindfulness'. *International Journal of Yoga Therapy,* 23(2): 15–24. doi: 10.17761/ijyt.23.2.r8735770101m8277

Egenes, L. and Reddy, K. (2016) *The Ramayana: A new retelling of Valmiki's ancient epic – complete and comprehensive.* New York: Penguin Random House.

Einstein, A. (1954) *Ideas and Opinions.* London: Crown.

Emerson, D. (2015) *Trauma-Sensitive Yoga in Therapy: bringing the body into treatment.* London: W. W. Norton and Company.

Enders, G. (2015) *Gut: the Inside Story of Our Most Underrated Organ.* London: Scribe.

Epstein, M. (2018) *Advice not Given.* London: Hay House UK Ltd.

Farhi, D. (2000) *Yoga Mind, Body and Spirit.* Dublin: Newleaf.

Farhi, D. (1996) *The Breathing Book.* New York: Henry Holt and Company.

Fogel, A. (2009) *The Psychophysiology of Self-Awareness: Rediscovering the Lost Art of Body Sense.* New York: W. W. Norton and Company.

Fogel, A. (2009) *Body Sense: The Science and Practice of Embodied Self-awareness.* New York: W. W. Norton and Company.

Bibliography

Forbes, B. (2011) *Yoga for Emotional Balance: Simple Practices to Help Relieve Anxiety and Depression.* Boston and London: Shambala.

Fosha, D., Siegel, D. J. and Solomon, M. D. (eds) (2009) *The Healing Power of Emotion: Affective Neuroscience, Development and Clinical Practice.* New York: W. W. Norton and Company.

Frank, R. (2005) 'Developmental Somatic Psychotherapy: Developmental Process Embodied within the Clinical Movement'. In Totton, N. (ed.) (2005), *New Dimensions in Body Psychotherapy.* Berkshire: Open University Press/McGraw-Hill Education.

Frank, R. and La Barre, F. (2011) *The First Year and the Rest of your Life: Movement, Development and Psychotherapeutic Change.* New York/London: Routledge.

Frankl, V. E. (1959) *Man's Search for Meaning.* London: Random House, 2004.

Freud, S. (2003 translation) *Beyond the Pleasure Principle and Other Writings.* London: Penguin.

Gallese, V., Fadiga, L., Fogassi, L. and Rizzolatti, G. (1996) 'Action Recognition in the Premotor Cortex'. *Brain*, 119, 593–609.

Gallese, V., Eagle, M. N. and Migone, P. (2007) 'Intentional Attunement: Mirror Neurons and the Neural Underpinnings of Interpersonal Relations'. *Journal of the American Psychoanalytic Association*, 55(1) 131–176.

Gendlin, E. (1978) *Focusing: How To Gain Direct Access To Your Body's Knowledge.* London: Rider.

Gerbarg, P. L. (2008) 'Yoga and Neuro-Psychoanalysis'. In Anderson, F. S. (ed.) (2008) *Bodies in Treatment: The Unspoken Dimension.* New York: The Analytic Press.

Gerbarg et al. (2011) 'Mass disasters and mind-body solutions: Evidence and Field Insights'. *Journal of the International Association of Yoga Therapists* 2(21): 23–34.

Gerhardt, S.(2004) *Why Love Matters: how affection shapes a baby's brain.* Hove: Routledge.

Gilbert, P. (2009) *The Compassionate Mind.* London: Robinson.

Gothe, Neha P., Khan, Imadh, Hayes, Jessica, Erlenbach, Emily and Damoiseaux, Jessica S. (2019) 'Yoga Effects on Brain Health: A

Systematic Review of the Current Literature.' *Brain Plasticity.* doi: 10.3233/BPL-190084

Grepmair, L., Mitterlehner, F., Loew, T., Bachler, E., Rother, W. and Nickel, M. (2007) 'Promoting Mindfulness in Psychotherapists in training influences the treatment results of their patients: A Randomised Double-Blind, Controlled Study'. *Psychotherapy and Psychosomatics* 2007; 76:332–8. doi: 10.1159/000107560

Harris, A. and Sinsheimer, K. (2008) 'The Analyst's Vulnerability: Preserving and Fine Tuning Analytic Bodies'. In Anderson, F. S. (ed.) (2008) *Bodies in Treatment: The Unspoken Dimension.* New York: The Analytic Press.

Harris, J. (2001) *Jung and Yoga: The Psyche–Body Connection.* Toronto: Inner City Books.

Hartley, L. (1995,1989) *Wisdom of the Body Moving: An introduction to Body-Mind Centering.* Berkeley, CA: North Atlantic Books.

Hatfield, E., Cacioppo, J. T. and Rapson, R. L. (1994) *Emotional Contagion: Studies in Emotion and Social Interaction.* Cambridge: Cambridge University Press.

Herman, J. (1992,1997) *Trauma and Recovery.* New York: Basic Books.

Holt-Lunstad, J., Smith, T. B. and Layton, J. B. (2010) 'Social Relationships and Mortality Risk: a meta-analytic review'. *PLOS Medicine.* doi: 10.1371/journal.pmed.1000316

Holt-Lunstad, J., Smith, T. B., Baker, M. and Harris, T. (2015) 'Loneliness and Isolation as Risk Factors for Mortality: a meta-analytic review'. *Perspectives on Psychological Science: a Journal for the Association of Psychological Science.* 2015, Mar; 10(2):227–37.

Holzel, B. K., Carmody, J., Congleton, C., Yerramsetti, S. M., Gardv and T., Lazar, S. W. (2011) 'Mindfulness practices lead to increases in regional brain gray matter density'. *Psychiatry Research: Neuroimaging Journal,* 191(1): 36–43.

Hrynchak, D. and Fouts G. (1998) 'Perception of Affect Attunement by Adolescents'. *Journal of Adolescence,* 21(1), 43–8.

Iyengar, B. K. S. (2005, 1966) *Light on Yoga.* New Delhi: Harper Collins.

Iyengar, B. K. S. (2019, 2005) *Light on Life: The journey to wholeness, inner peace and ultimate freedom.* London: Rodale International Ltd.

Bibliography

Johnson, S. M. (1994) *Character Styles*. New York: W. W. Norton and Company.

Jung, C. G. (1963) *Memories, Dreams, Reflections*. London: Collins and Routledge and Kegan Paul.

Kahneman, D., Diener, E. and Schwartz, N. (1999) *Well-being: the Foundations of Hedonic Psychology*. Russell Sage Foundation.

Kaminoff, L. (2007) *Yoga Anatomy*. Leeds: Human Kinetics.

Kandel, E. R. (2006) *In Search of Memory: The Emergence of a New Science of Mind*. New York: W. W. Norton and Company.

Khalsa, S. B. (2004) 'Yoga as a Therapeutic Intervention: a Bibliometric Analysis of Published Research Studies'. *Indian Journal of Physiology and Pharmacology*, 2004, July; 48(3): 269–85.

Kirkwood, G. et al. (2005) 'Yoga for Anxiety: A Systematic Review of the Research Evidence'. *British Journal of Sports Medicine* 2005, Dec.; 39: 884–91. www.pubmedcentral.nih.gov/articlerender.fcgi?artid=1725091&tool=pmcentrez&rendertype=abstract

Kjaer, T. W., Bertelson, C., Piccin, P., Brooks, D., Alving, J. and Lou, H. C. (2002) 'Increased Dopamine tone during meditation-induced change of consciousness'. *Cognitive Brain Research*, vol 13, issue 2, April 2002: 255–9. doi: 10.1016/S0926-6410(01)00106-9

Klein, M. (1932, 1997) *The Psycho-analysis of Children*. London: Vintage

Kohut, H.(1977) *The Restoration of the Self*. Chicago: University of Chicago Press.

Kraftsow, G. (2002) *Yoga for Transformation*. London: Penguin Books.

Lowen, A. (1975) *Bioenergetics: The revolutionary therapy that uses the language of the body to heal the problems of the mind*. Arkana: Penguin.

Lutz, A., McFarlin, D., Perlman, D., Salmons, T. and Davidson, R. (2013) 'Altered anterior insula activation during anticipation and experience of painful stimuli in expert meditators'. *Neuroimage*, 64: 538–46.

Majewski, L. and Balayogi Bhavanani, A. (2020). *Yoga Therapy as a Whole-Person Approach to Health*. London: Singing Dragon.

Mate, G. (2019) *When the Body Says No: The Cost of Hidden Stress*. London: Penguin Random House.

McGilchrist, I. (2009) *The Master and His Emissary: the divided brain and the making of the western world*. New Haven: Yale University Press.

Merleau-Ponty, M. (1962) *The Phenomenology of Perception*. London: Routledge and Kegan-Paul.

Michalsen, A. et al. (2005) 'Rapid Stress Reduction and Anxiolysis Among Distressed Women as a Consequence of a Three-Month Intensive Yoga Program'. *Medical Science Monitor* 11(12): 555–61.

Muir, J. (1911) *My First Summer in the Sierra*. Cambridge: Riverside Press.

Neff, K. and Germer, C. (2018) *The Mindful Self-Compassion Workbook*. London: Guildford Press.

Ogden, P., Minton, K. and Pain, C. (2006) *Trauma and the Body*. New York: W. W. Norton and Company.

Panksepp, J. (1998) *Affective Neuroscience: the Foundations of Human and Animal Emotions*. Oxford: Oxford University Press.

Payne, H. and Warnecke, T. (2013) Editorial. *Body, Movement and Dance in Psychotherapy: An International Journal for Theory, Research and Practice*, vol 8(1): 1–4

Pert, C. B. (1997) *Molecules of Emotion: Why You Feel the Way You Feel*. London: Simon and Schuster.

Pilkington, K. et al. (2005) 'Yoga for Depression: The Research Evidence.' *Journal of Affective Disorders*, 89: 13–24.

Porges, S. W. (2003) 'The Polyvagal theory: phylogenetic contributions to social behavior'. *Physiology and Behavior*, 79 (2003): 503–13.

Porges, S. W. (2009) 'Reciprocal Influences Between Body and Brain in the Perception and Expression of Affect: A Polyvagal Perspective.' In Siegel, D. J., Solomon, M., Fosha, D. (eds) (2009) *The Healing Power of Emotion: Affective Neuroscience, Development, and Clinical Practice*. New York and London: Norton and Co.

Rhodes, A. M. (2014) *Yoga for Traumatic Stress* (Dissertation: Boston College), in Emerson (2015).

Ross, A. and Michalsen, A. (2016) 'Yoga for Prevention and Wellness'. In Khalsa, S. B. S., Cohen, L., McCall, T. and Telles, S. (eds) *The Principles and Practice of Yoga in Healthcare*. Pencaitland: Handspring Publishing, 473.

Bibliography

Rothschild, B. (2000) *The Body Remembers: The Psychophysiology of Trauma and Trauma Treatment.* London and New York: Norton.

Rothschild, B. (2006) *Help for the Helper.* New York Norton.

Satchidananda, S. (2009) *The Yoga Sutras of Patanjali.* Virginia: Integral Yoga Publications.

Scaravelli, V. (1991) *Awakening the Spine.* New York: Labyrinth Publishing.

Schore, A. N. (1994) *Affect Regulation and the Origin of the Self.* Hillsdale, NJ: Erlbaum.

Schore, A. N. (2012) *The Science of the Art of Psychotherapy.* New York: Norton.

Shaw, R. (2003) *The Embodied Psychotherapist: The Therapist's Body Story.* Hove and New York: Brunner Routledge.

Siegel, D. J. (1999) *The Developing Mind: Toward a Neurobiology of Interpersonal Experience.* New York: Guildford.

Siegel, D. J. and Schore, A. N. (2009) Preface to Norton Series on interpersonal neurobiology in Fogel, A. (2009) *The Psychophysiology of Self-Awareness: Rediscovering the Lost Art of Body Sense.* New York: W. W. Norton and Company.

Siegel, D. J. (2010) *The Mindful Therapist.* New York: W. W. Norton and Company.

Siegel, D. J. (2010) *Mindsight: Transform your brain with the new science of kindness.* London: Random House.

Siegman, A. F. et al. 'Antagonistic Behaviour, Dominance, Hostility, and Coronary Heart Disease'. *Psychosomatic Medicine* 62 (2000), 248–57.

Simon, N. M., Hofmann, G. S., Rosenfield D., Hoeppner, S. S., Hoge, E. A., Bui, E. and Khalsa S. B. S. 'Efficacy of Yoga vs Cognitive Behavioral Therapy vs Stress Education for the Treatment of Generalized Anxiety Disorder: A Randomized Clinical Trial'. *JAMA Psychiatry* 2021; 78(1): 13–20. doi: 10.1001/jamapsychiatry.2020.2496

Sovick, R. (1999) 'The Science of Breathing: the Yogic View in Progress'. *Brain Research,* 122: 491–505.

Stamenov, M. and Gallese, V. (eds) (2002) *Mirror Neurons and the Evolution of Brain and Language.* Philadelphia: John Benjamins.

Stern, D. N. (1985) *The Interpersonal World of the Infant*. New York: Basic Books.

Stern, D. N. (2003) *Unformulated Experience: From Dissociation to Imagination in Psychoanalysis*. Hillsdale, NJ: Analytic Press.

Stern, D. N. (2004) *The Present Moment in Psychotherapy and Everyday Life*. New York: W. W. Norton and Company.

Stone, M. (2006) 'The analyst's body as tuning fork: embodied resonance in countertransference'. *Journal of Analytical Psychology*, 51:109–24.

Streeter, C. et al. (2012) 'Effects of Yoga on the Autonomic Nervous System, Gamma-aminobutryic-acid, and Allostasis in Epilepsy, Depression, and Post-traumatic Stress Disorder'. *Medical Hypotheses*, 78(5): 571–9.

Suzuki, S. (1970) *Zen Mind, Beginner's Mind: informal talks on Zen meditation and practice*. Boulder, Colorado: Shambala Publications.

Swami Muktibodhananda (1985, 1998) *Hatha Yoga Pradipika: light on hatha yoga*. Bihar, India: Yoga Publications Trust.

Swami Rama, Ballentine, R., Swami Ajaya. (1976) *Yoga and Psychotherapy: the evolution of consciousness*. Honesdale, Pennsylvania: The Himalayan International Institute of Yoga Science and Philosophy.

Swami Rama (1985) *Perennial Psychology of the Bhagavad Gita*. Honesdale, Pennsylvania: The Himalayan International Institute of Yoga Science and Philosophy.

Swami Satyananda Saraswati (1969, 2008) *Asana Pranayama Mudra Bandha*. Bihar, India: Yoga Publications Trust.

Telles et al. (2012) 'Managing Mental Health Disorders Resulting from Trauma Through Yoga: A Review'. *Depression Research and Treatment*, Article ID 401513, 9 pages. doi: 10.1155/2012/401513

Totton, N. and Edmonson, E. (2009) *Reichian Growth Work*. Ross on Wye: PCCS.

Trevarthen, C. (1993) 'The Self Born in Intersubjectivity: an Infant Communicating', in Neisser, U. (ed.), *The Perceived Self* (121–73). New York: Cambridge University Press.

Bibliography

Tyagi, A. and Cohen, M. 'Yoga and Heart Rate Variability: A systematic review of the literature'. *International Journal of Yoga,* 2016, July–Dec; 9(2): 97–103.

Upadhyay-Dhungel, K. and Sohal, A. 'Physiology of nostril breathing exercises and its probable relation with nostril and cerebral dominance: a theoretical research on literature'. *Janaki Medical College Journal of Medical Science,* vol 1, 1, 2013, doi: 10.3126/jmcjm.v1i1.7885

Valente, V. G. and Marotta, A. (2005) 'The impact of yoga on the professional and personal life of the psychotherapist'. *Contemporary Family Therapy* 27(1): 65–80.

Valente, V. G. and Marotta, A. (2011) 'Prescribing Yoga to Supplement and Support Psychotherapy'. In McMinn J. et al. (eds) *Spiritually Oriented Interventions for Counselling and Psychotherapy,* 251–76. Washington: American Psychological Association.

Van der Kolk, B. (1994) 'The Body Keeps The Score: Memory and the Evolving Psychobiology of Post-Traumatic Stress'. *Harvard Review of Psychiatry* 1(5): 253–65.

Van der Kolk, B. (2006) 'Clinical Implications of Neuroscience Research in PTSD'. *Annals of the New York Academy of Sciences.* doi: 10.1196/annals.1364.022

Van der Kolk, B. (2014) 'Yoga as an Adjunctive Therapy for PTSD'. *Journal of Clinical Psychiatry,* 75: no 6: 559–65.

Van der Kolk, B. (2014, Kindle Edition) *The Body Keeps The Score: Mind, Brain and Body in the Transformation of Trauma.* London: Penguin.

Weintraub, A. (2004). *Yoga for Depression: A compassionate guide to relieve suffering through yoga.* New York: Broadway Books, Random House.

West, J. (2011) *Moving to Heal: Women's Experience of Therapeutic Yoga after Complex Trauma.* PhD dissertation, Boston College.

Winnicott, D. W. (1965) *The Maturational Processes and the Facilitating Environment.* London: Hogarth Press.

Young, C. (2012) *About the Science of Body Psychotherapy.* Galashiels: Body Psychotherapy Publications.

Notes

Introduction
1   Muir, J. (1911) *My First Summer in the Sierra*. Cambridge: Riverside Press.

Chapter One
2   Balasubramaniam, M. et al. (2012) 'Yoga on our Minds: a Systematic Review of Yoga for Neuropsychiatric Disorders'. *Frontiers in Psychiatry*. Pre-published online 12 October 2012. doi: 10.3389/fpsyt.2012.00117; Becker, I. (2008) 'Uses of Yoga in Psychiatry and Medicine'. *Complementary and Alternative Medicine and Psychiatry*, vol 19: 107–42; Valente, V. G. and Marotta, A. (2011) 'Prescribing Yoga to Supplement and Support Psychotherapy'. In McMinn J. et al. (eds) *Spiritually Oriented Interventions for Counselling and Psychotherapy*, 251–76. Washington: American Psychological Association; Davidson, R. J. and Kabat-Zinn, J. (2003) 'Alterations in Brain and Immune Function Produced by Mindfulness Meditation'. *Psychosomatic Medicine* 65(4): 564–70; Forbes, B. (2011) *Yoga for Emotional Balance: Simple Practices to Help Relieve Anxiety and Depression*. Boston and London: Shambala; Gerberg, P. L. (2008) 'Yoga and Neuro-Psychoanalysis'. In Anderson, F. S. (ed.) (2008) *Bodies in Treatment: The Unspoken Dimension*. New York: The Analytic Press; Holzel, B. K., Carmody, J., Congleton, C., Yerramsetti, S. M., Gardv, T. and Lazar, S. W. (2011) 'Mindfulness practices lead to increases in regional brain gray matter density'. *Psychiatry Research: Neuroimaging Journal*, 191(1): 36–43; Khalsa, S. B. (2004) 'Yoga as a Therapeutic Intervention: a Bibliometric Analysis of Published Research Studies'. *Indian Journal of Physiology and Pharmacology*, 2004, July; 48(3): 269–85.
Kirkwood, G. et al. (2005) 'Yoga for Anxiety: A Systematic Review of the Research Evidence'. *British Journal of Sports Medicine*, 2005, Dec; 39: 884–91; Kirkwood, G. et al. (2005) 'Yoga for Anxiety: A

Notes

Systematic Review of the Research Evidence'. *British Journal of Sports Medicine* 2005, Dec; 39: 884–91; Lutz, A., McFarlin, D., Perlman, D., Salmons, T. and Davidson, R. (2013) 'Altered anterior insula activation during anticipation and experience of painful stimuli in expert meditators'. *Neuroimage,* 64: 538–46; Michalsen, A. et al. (2005). 'Rapid Stress Reduction and Anxiolysis Among Distressed Women as a Consequence of a Three-Month Intensive Yoga Program'. *Medical Science Monitor* 11(12): 555–61; Sovick, R. (1999) 'The Science of Breathing: the Yogic View in Progress'. *Brain Research,* 122: 491–505; Streeter, C. et al. (2012) 'Effects of Yoga on the Autonomic Nervous System, Gamma-aminobutryic-acid, and Allostasis in Epilepsy, Depression, and Post-traumatic Stress Disorder'. *Medical Hypotheses,* 78(5): 571–9; Telles et al. (2012) 'Managing Mental Health Disorders Resulting from Trauma Through Yoga: A Review'. *Depression Research and Treatment,* Article ID 401513, 9 pages. doi: 10.1155/2012/401513.

3 Brisbon, N. M. and Lowery, G. A. (2011) 'Mindfulness and Levels of Stress: A comparison of beginner and advanced hatha yoga practitioners'. *Journal of Religion and Health,* 50, no.4, 931–41. doi: 10.1007/s10943-009 9305-3; Brown, R. P. and Gerbarg, P. L. (2009) 'Yoga Breathing, Meditation and Longevity'. *Annals of the New York Academy of Sciences* 1172, 54–62. doi: 10.1111/j.1749-6632.2009.04394.x

Chapter Two

4 Simon, N. M., Hofmann, G. S., Rosenfield D., Hoeppner, S. S., Hoge, E. A. Bui, E. and Khalsa, S. B. S. 'Efficacy of Yoga vs Cognitive Behavioral Therapy vs Stress Education for the Treatment of Generalized Anxiety Disorder: A Randomized Clinical Trial'. *JAMA Psychiatry* 2021; 78(1): 13–20. doi: 10.1001/jamapsychiatry.2020.2496; Streeter, C. et al. (2012) 'Effects of Yoga on the Autonomic Nervous System, Gamma-aminobutryic-acid, and Allostasis in Epilepsy, Depression, and Post-traumatic Stress Disorder'. *Medical Hypotheses,* 78(5): 571–9; Michalsen, A. et al. (2005). 'Rapid Stress Reduction and Anxiolysis Among Distressed Women as a Consequence of a Three-Month Intensive Yoga Program'. *Medical Science Monitor* 11(12): 555–61;

Kirkwood, G. et al. (2005) 'Yoga for Anxiety: A Systematic Review of the Research Evidence'. *British Journal of Sports Medicine* 2005, Dec; 39: 884–91; Khalsa, S. B. (2004) 'Yoga as a Therapeutic Intervention: a Bibliometric Analysis of Published Research Studies'. *Indian Journal of Physiology and Pharmacology,* 2004, July; 48(3): 269–85.
5. Gothe, Neha P., Khan, Imadh, Hayes, Jessica, Erlenbach, Emily, Damoiseaux and Jessica S. (2019) 'Yoga Effects on Brain Health: A Systematic Review of the Current Literature.' *Brain Plasticity.* doi: 10.3233/BPL-190084

Chapter Three
6. Satchidananda, Swami (2009) *The Yoga Sutras of Patanjali.* Virginia: Integral Yoga Publications.

Chapter Four
7. Rogers, C. (1951) *Client-centered Therapy: Its current practice, implications and theory.* London: Constable.
8. Neff, K. and Germer, C., (2018) *The Mindful Self-Compassion Workbook.* London: Guildford Press.
9. Boellinghaus, I., Jones, F. W. and Hutton, J. (2014) 'The Role of Mindfulness and Loving-kindness Meditation in Cultivating Self-compassion and Other-focused Concern in Health Care Professionals'. *Mindfulness* 5, 129–38. doi: 10.1007/s12671-012-0158-6

Chapter Five
10. Hatfield, E., Cacioppo, J. T. and Rapson, R. L. (1994) *Emotional Contagion: Studies in Emotion and Social Interaction.* Cambridge: Cambridge University Press.
11. Cozolino, L. (2002, 2017) *The Neuroscience of Psychotherapy: Healing the Social Brain.* London: W. W. Norton and Company.
Cozolino, (2006, 2014) *The Neuroscience of Human Relationships: Attachment and the Developing Social Brain.* London: W. W. Norton and Company.
12. Twitter, 28 September 2020.

Notes

13 Dunn, K. D. (2008) 'A review of the literature examining the physiological processes underlying the therapeutic benefits of Hatha yoga'. *Adv Mind Body Med*, 2008, September; 23 (3):10–8; Farhi, D. (1996) *The Breathing Book*. New York: Henry Holt and Company; Majewski, L. and Balayogi Bhavanani, A. (2020). *Yoga Therapy as a Whole-Person Approach to Health*. London: Singing Dragon; Sovick, R. (1999) 'The Science of Breathing: the Yogic View in Progress'. *Brain Research*, 122: 491–505; Ross, A. and Michalsen, A. (2016) 'Yoga for Prevention and Wellness'. In Khalsa, S. B. S., Cohen, L., McCall, T. and Telles, S. (eds) *The Principles and Practice of Yoga in Healthcare*. Pencaitland: Handspring Publishing, 473; Devasena, I., Narhare, P. (2011) 'Effect of yoga on heart rate and blood pressure and its clinical significance'. *International Journal of Biological and Medical Research*, 2011; 2(3):75–753.

Chapter Six

14 Bowlby, J. (1969) *Attachment and Loss*. London: Random House.
15 Tyagi, A., Cohen, M. 'Yoga and Heart Rate Variability: A systematic review of the literature'. *International Journal of Yoga*, 2016, July–Dec; 9(2):97–103
16 Porges, S. W. (2003) 'The Polyvagal theory: phylogenetic contributions to social behavior'. *Physiology and Behavior* 79 (2003): 503–513; Porges, S. W. (2009) 'Reciprocal Influences Between Body and Brain in the Perception and Expression of Affect: A Polyvagal Perspective'. In Siegel, D. J., Solomon, M. and Fosha, D. (eds) (2009) *The Healing Power of Emotion: Affective Neuroscience, Development, and Clinical Practice*. NY, London: Norton and Co.

Chapter Nine

17 Winnicott, D. W. (1965) *The Maturational Processes and the Facilitating Environment*. London: Hogarth Press.

Chapter Ten

18 Klein, M. (1932, 1997) *The Psycho-analysis of Children*. London: Vintage.
19 Jung, C. G. (1963) *Memories, Dreams, Reflections*. London: Collins and Routledge and Kegan Paul.

20 Suzuki, S. (1970) *Zen Mind, Beginner's Mind: informal talks on Zen meditation and practice.* Boulder, Colorado Shambala Publications.

Chapter Eleven

21 Bion, W. R. (1970) *Attention and Interpretation.* London: Tavistock Publications Ltd.
22 Craig, A. D. (2010) 'The Sentient Self'. *Brain Structure and Function,* 214(5–6): 563–77.
23 Van der Kolk, B. (1994) 'The Body Keeps The Score: Memory and the Evolving Psychobiology of Post-Traumatic Stress'. *Harvard Review of Psychiatry* 1(5): 253–65; Van der Kolk, B. (2006) 'Clinical Implications of Neuroscience Research in PTSD'. *Annals of the New York Academy of Sciences.* doi: 10.1196/annals.1364.022; Van der Kolk, B. (2014) 'Yoga as an Adjunctive Therapy for PTSD'. *Journal of Clinical Psychiatry,* 75: no 6: 559–65; Van der Kolk, B. (2014, Kindle Edition) *The Body Keeps The Score: Mind, Brain and Body in the Transformation of Trauma.* London: Penguin.
24 Damasio, A. (1999) *The Feeling of What Happens: Body and Emotion in the Making of Consciousness.* New York: Hartcourt Bruce.
25 Damasio, A. (1994) *Descartes' Error: Emotion, Reason and the Human Brain.* New York: Penguin.
26 Pert, C. B. (1997) *Molecules of Emotion: Why You Feel the Way You Feel.* London: Simon and Schuster.
27 Porges, S. W. (2003) 'The Polyvagal theory: phylogenetic contributions to social behavior'. *Physiology and Behavior,* 79 (2003): 503–13; Porges, S. W. (2009) 'Reciprocal Influences Between Body and Brain in the Perception and Expression of Affect: A Polyvagal Perspective'. In Siegel, D. J., Solomon, M. and Fosha, D. (eds) (2009) *The Healing Power of Emotion: Affective Neuroscience, Development, and Clinical Practice.* NY, London: Norton and Co.

Chapter Twelve

28 Freud, S. (2003 translation) *Beyond the Pleasure Principle and Other Writings.* London: Penguin.

Notes

29. Kahneman, D., Diener, E. and Schwartz, N. (1999) *Well-being: the Foundations of Hedonic Psychology*. Russell Sage Foundation.
30. Fogel, A. (2009) *The Psychophysiology of Self-Awareness: Rediscovering the Lost Art of Body Sense*. New York: W. W. Norton and Company; Fogel, A. (2009) *Body Sense: The Science and Practice of Embodied Self-awareness*. New York: W. W. Norton and Company; Panksepp, J. (1998) *Affective Neuroscience: the Foundations of Human and Animal Emotions*. Oxford: Oxford University Press; Fosha, D., Siegel, D. J. and Solomon, M. D. (eds) (2009) *The Healing Power of Emotion: Affective Neuroscience, Development and Clinical Practice*. New York: W. W. Norton and Company.
31. Frankl, V. E. (1959) *Man's Search for Meaning*. London: Random House, 2004.
32. Davidson, R. J. and Kabat-Zinn, J. (2003) 'Alterations in Brain and Immune Function Produced by Mindfulness Meditation'. *Psychosomatic Medicine* 65(4): 564–70; Holzel, B. K., Carmody, J., Congleton, C., Yerramsetti, S. M., Gardv, T. and Lazar, S. W. (2011) 'Mindfulness practices lead to increases in regional brain gray matter density'. *Psychiatry Research: Neuroimaging Journal*, 191(1): 36–43.

Chapter Thirteen

33. Armstrong, J. and Rishi, K. (2020) *The Bhagavad Gita Comes Alive: A radical translation*. Vancouver: VASA Publishing.

Chapter Fourteen

34. Siegman, A. F. et al. 'Antagonistic Behaviour, Dominance, Hostility, and Coronary Heart Disease'. *Psychosomatic Medicine* 62 (2000), 248–57.
35. Mate, G. (2019) *When the Body Says No: The Cost of Hidden Stress*. London: Penguin Random House.
36. Iyengar, B. K. S. (2005, 1966) *Light on Yoga*. New Delhi: Harper Collins.

Chapter Fifteen

37. Suzuki, S. (1970) *Zen Mind, Beginner's Mind: informal talks on Zen meditation and practice*. Boulder, Colorado: Shambala Publications.

Chapter Sixteen

38 Mate, G. (2019) *When the Body Says No: The Cost of Hidden Stress.* London: Penguin Random House.
39 Siegel, D. J. (1999) *The Developing Mind: Toward a Neurobiology of Interpersonal Experience.* New York: Guildford.
40 Mate, G. (2019) *When the Body Says No: The Cost of Hidden Stress.* London: Penguin Random House.
41 Streeter, C. C., Jensen, J. E., Perlmutter, R. M., Cabral, H. J., Hua Tian Terhune, D. B., Ciraulo, D. A. and Renshwaw, P. F. (2007). 'Yoga asana sessions increase brain GABA levels'. Pilot study in the *Journal of Alternative and Complementary Medicine*, vol 13, no. 4. Published online 28 May 2007. doi: 10.1089/acm.2007.6338

Chapter Eighteen

42 The Campaign to End Loneliness.
43 Holt-Lunstad, J., Smith, T. B. and Layton, J. B (2010) 'Social Relationships and Mortality Risk: a meta-analytic review'. *PLOS Medicine.* doi: 10.1371/journal.pmed.1000316; Holt-Lunstad, J., Smith, T. B., Baker, M., Harris, T. (2015) 'Loneliness and Isolation as Risk Factors for Mortality: a meta-analytic review'. *Perspectives on Psychological Science: a Journal for the Association of Psychological Science.* 2015, Mar.; 10(2): 227–37.
44 Kohut, H.(1977) *The Restoration of the Self.* Chicago: University of Chicago Press.
45 McGilchrist, I. (2009) *The Master and His Emissary: the Divided Brain and the Making of the Western World.* place? Yale University Press.
46 Upadhyay-Dhungel, K., Sohal, A. 'Physiology of nostril breathing exercises and its probable relation with nostril and cerebral dominance: a theoretical research on literature'. *Janaki Medical College Journal of Medical Science,* vol 1, 1, 2013. doi: 10.3126/jmcjm.v1i1.7885

Chapter Nineteen

47 Gallese, V., Fadiga, L., Fogassi, L. and Rizzolatti, G. (1996) 'Action Recognition in the Premotor Cortex'. *Brain*, 119, 593–609; Gallese,V., Eagle, M. N. and Migone, P. (2007) 'Intentional Attunement: Mirror Neurons

Notes

and the Neural Underpinnings of Interpersonal Relations'. *Journal of the American Psychoanalytic Association*, 55(1) 1310–176; Hatfield, E., Cacioppo, J. T. and Rapson, R. L. (1994) *Emotional Contagion: Studies in Emotion and Social Interaction.* Cambridge: Cambridge University Press; Pert, C. B. (1997) *Molecules of Emotion: Why You Feel the Way You Feel.* London: Simon and Schuster; Schore, A. N. (1994) *Affect Regulation and the Origin of the Self.* Hillsdale, NJ: Erlbaum; Schore, A. N. (2012) *The Science of the Art of Psychotherapy.* New York: Norton; Siegel, D. J. (1999) *The Developing Mind: Toward a Neurobiology of Interpersonal Experience.* New York: Guildford; Siegel, D. J. and Schore, A. N. (2009) Preface to Norton Series on interpersonal neurobiology in Fogel, A. (2009) *The Psychophysiology of Self-Awareness: Rediscovering the Lost Art of Body Sense.* New York: W. W. Norton and Company; Siegel, D. J. (2010) *The Mindful Therapist.* New York: W. W. Norton and Company; Stamenov, M. and Gallese, V. (eds) (2002) *Mirror Neurons and the Evolution of Brain and Language.* Philadelphia: John Benjamins.

48 Stern, D. N. (1985) *The Interpersonal World of the Infant.* New York: Basic Books; Stern, D. N. (2003) *Unformulated Experience: From Dissociation to Imagination in Psychoanalysis.* Hillsdale, NJ: Analytic Press; Stern, D. N. (2004) *The Present Moment in Psychotherapy and Everyday Life.* New York: W. W. Norton and Company; Trevarthen, C. (1993) 'The Self Born in Intersubjectivity: an Infant Communicating', in Neisser, U. (ed.), *The Perceived Self* (121–73). New York: Cambridge University Press; Winnicott, D. W. (1965) *The Maturational Processes and the Facilitating Environment.* London: Hogarth Press.

49 Kjaer, T. W., Bertelson, C., Piccin, P., Brooks, D., Alving, J. and Lou, H. C. (2002) 'Increased Dopamine tone during meditation-induced change of consciousness'. *Cognitive Brain Research*, vol 13, issue 2, April 2002: 255–259. doi: 10.1016/S0926-6410(01)00106-9

Chapter Twenty

50 Bromberg, P. M. (1996) 'Standing in the spaces: The multiplicity of self and the psychoanalytic relationship'. *Contemporary Psychoanalysis*, 32(4), 509–35.

Acknowledgements

I have had many, many teachers over the years and would like to give heartfelt thanks to all of them.

To those from the institutions who provided me with such good trainings – The Minster Centre where I trained as a psychotherapist, Yogamind Australia who provided my first yoga teacher training and to Yogacampus who provided my second yoga teacher training.

To the individual teachers I have known, loved, learned, and continue to learn from: Catherine Annis, Chloe Fremantle, Wade Gotwals, Jean Hall, Rachel Johnston, Liz Lark, Aki Omori, Karen Russell, Freddie Sardais, Liz Warrington and Zephyr Wildman.

To the friends who have supported me by reading drafts of this book and providing such invaluable feedback – Sandra Gillespie, Inge Samuels and Nicole Scott.

To Lee Watson and all the members of the Fierce Calm community who have shared their stories so generously.

To all the yogic teachers and sages through the ages who have developed, evolved, codified and transmitted what they have discovered about such a transformative practice – one which has meant so much to so many. And to all the psychotherapeutic practitioners, theorists and writers who have similarly studied and learned and developed the equally transformative practice of psychotherapy.

To all my therapy clients and yoga students who have shared their stories and their journeys with me and allowed me to learn from them.

Acknowledgements

To my agent, Jane Graham Maw, my editor, Jacqui Lewis, and to all at Yellow Kite.

Thank you all so very much.

All mistakes and any clumsiness of thought or language are very much my own.

About the Author

Sasha Bates is a former filmmaker turned psychotherapist, author and yoga teacher. She first found yoga in her early twenties, seeking a cure for insomnia and stress. She entered psychotherapy at this time too, finding that both these new discoveries provided her alternative ways of understanding herself and healthier ways of relating to herself, and to others. As she moved through researching, directing and series producing on shows as diverse as *Watchdog*, *Live and Kicking*, *Omnibus*, *Grand Designs* and *How to Look Good Naked*, she found the joy and interest in her television world began to pall. She found solace by diving deeper into the twin pillars of support – yoga and therapy – that had sustained her throughout her two absorbing, if stressful, decades in the media.

Wanting to know more about each discipline, she started training to be both a yoga teacher and a psychotherapist. The more she delved into, the more she read about, the more she practised both, the more she saw parallels. This led to her writing her MA thesis on the multitude of overlaps that she found between the two, and concluding that massive benefits could result from practising both – for clients and therapists alike.

Leaving the world of television behind, Sasha went on to teach yoga in gyms and studios, in corporations and privately, all while also working as a psychotherapist within NHS and higher-education institutions. Setting up her own private psychotherapeutic practice, she found herself using all that she knew from her long years of yoga practice as both student and teacher to further

About the Author

enrich the work she did with her therapy clients. The two disciplines led to further training in Trauma Sensitive Yoga.

All this study and practice proved invaluable in Sasha's own life when her world was shaken to its core with the unexpected death of her husband, Bill, at just fifty-six. She also turned back to writing, hoping to make sense of the tumultuous feelings of grief that were overwhelming her. As she wrote her pain down onto the page, she began to find her 'therapist self' entering the conversation, trying to use what she knew of therapeutic theory to help navigate through the new and unwelcome world into which she had been thrust. The resulting book, *Languages of Loss*, part memoir, part psychoeducation delves into what therapeutic wisdom can offer grievers. Her second book *A Grief Companion* – written in response to all the letters she received after the publication of *Languages of Loss* in the midst of the Covid pandemic – offers more practical suggestions as to how to navigate those painful first few months when everything is so raw and support feels hard to find.

In *Yoga Saved My Life* Sasha returns to her passion for exploring what yoga and psychotherapy together can offer those grappling with the big issues and concerns facing most of us today – anxiety, stress, depression, anger, conflict, addiction, uncertainty, loneliness and more.

Sasha continues her work as a journalist, psychotherapist and tutor. She teaches workshops about grief, yoga and self-regulation to other therapists, and to the general public. She has also founded a commemorative theatrical bursary she set up in honour of her late husband – The Bill Cashmore Award – in conjunction with The Lyric Theatre, Hammersmith.

To find out more and keep up to date with Sasha's workshops, please visit sashabates.co.uk

Follow @sashbates on Instagram, Twitter and Facebook.

Also by Sasha Bates

LANGUAGES OF LOSS
A psychotherapist's journey through grief

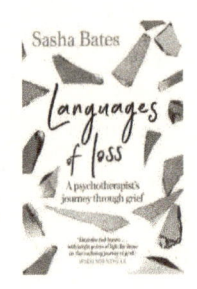

One person, two perspectives on grief. Plunged unexpectedly into widowhood at just 49 years old, psychotherapist Sasha Bates describes in searing honesty the agonisingly raw feelings unleashed by the loss of her husband and best friend, Bill. At the same time, she attempts to keep her therapist hat in place and create some perspective from psychoanalytic theory. From the depths of her confusion she gropes for ways to manage and bear the pain – by looking back at all that she has learned from psychotherapeutic research, and from accepted grief theories, to help her make sense of her altered reality.

Paperback 978 1 529 31716 9

A GRIEF COMPANION
Practical support and a guiding hand through the darkness of loss

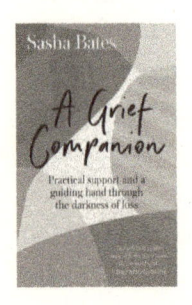

Split into four sections that can be read in any order – Mind, Body, Spirit and Everyday – this book explores the non-linear grief that you may be feeling and gives you permission to do your grief, your way. Filled with suggestions, resources, advice for friends of the bereaved and a guiding hand, this book will help you see some light in the darkness of grief.

Trade Paperback 978 1 529 34360 1

yellow kite

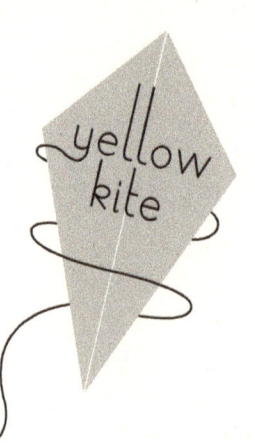

books to help you live a good life

Join the conversation and tell us how you live a #goodlife

@yellowkitebooks
YellowKiteBooks
Yellow Kite Books
YellowKiteBooks